THRIVING WITH RHEUMATOID ARTHRITIS

FROM SEX TO SOCKS: TIPS, HACKS & SHORTCUTS TO MAKE LIFE WITH RA EASIER

HELEN WARD DAY

BELLA LUNA
PRODUCTIONS

THRIVING WITH RHEUMATOID ARTHRITIS

CONTENTS

*To my husband, with special thanks
for his wonderful role as my helpmate.*

INTRODUCTION

During the week of my 40th birthday, I was diagnosed with
rheumatoid arthritis (RA). RA is an autoimmune disorder that
attacks the joints and causes painful swelling, inflammation,
and sometimes, immobility. It can also attack other parts of
your body from your skin to your brain.

Upon hearing it, my world tilted—like the feeling of going
too fast on an amusement ride. My brain was instantly
clogged with the terms my doctor was throwing at me while my
mind raced with endless possibilities. I wanted off this ride,
now.

What would this mean for my future, my plans? I had been
struggling with completing my daily activities for a while based
on other health problems I had going on at the time. But this
one, this diagnosis, was the exclamation point. It pinpoint-
ed the real reasons for my limited mobility. It told me there was
a tangible reason why I continued to decline in the activities I
was used to doing. My doctor and I both knew this diagnosis
was going to change my life and the way I maneuvered, thought
about and carried out my day-to-day activities.

As I was leaving, my doctor mentioned a thought that has

always lingered with me, even now with 15+ years of RA under my belt:

"A 'glass-half-empty-person' will always see the worst in every situation, and that's how you let an autoimmune disorder control your life. You have to see the glass half-full. Always."

After my appointment, I went out to my car and had a long, hard cry. But then I got mad. I was mad about all the doctors I'd visited in the previous ten years who had dismissed my symptoms. I was mad my new rheumatologist had asked me, "Why did you wait so long to come in and start treatment for this?" I was mad about a lot. But I didn't stay mad. I decided to channel anger into determination.

I wiped my eyes and immediately started to develop a plan for how I was going to tackle RA and all of its hindrances. I wouldn't let it defeat me.

Then, I decided on something audacious. I decided, at that moment, sitting in my chilly car, not only would I not become disabled—instead, I'd run a marathon.

My doctor was right. I had to be positive. I took my initial anger and turned it into determination to live well and live fully. The marathon would be a tangible, visible commitment to this. Then, I set out to work toward this goal to the best of my abilities.

I really wish I had words to describe for you the feeling of accomplishment of crossing the finish line of a marathon, with loved ones waiting for me, and cheering my last few steps.

But I can't. I have not run a marathon. But I have finished *three half marathons*. With the glass half-full viewpoint, you could say I exceeded my goal by 50%.

Now, don't get me wrong; there are many days where I'm not strong. RA is a disorder that continually attacks the synovial fluid surrounding the joints, and I have to be conscious that even when I'm not thinking about it, it's there.

I wake up some days and can't do the things I did the day

before. But the points I've decided to focus on are the ones that eliminate extra stress from my life. With all there is to enjoy and see in the world, why should I focus on the stress of not being able to open a pickle jar? Having RA drains precious energy from the body, and I would rather put what energy I have left into *living*.

As a former academic librarian, I've been writing peer-reviewed medical articles since 1997. My motivation to write this book is to share with others some of what I've learned along with my own personal experiences, which I will include in each chapter in this book. I have included hacks that I use in my day-to-day life, including cleaning and organizing my household, and a ton of tips I gleaned from others.

However, this book is not intended as medical advice. You should seek the advice of your doctor or other qualified medical practitioner before following any of the suggestions in this book.

Coming to terms with my diagnosis was only the beginning. RA is a chameleon—it changes day to day and week to week. But I can adapt day to day and week to week right along with it. Human beings are capable of learning throughout their lives. And when we can learn, we can adapt. Knowing you can adapt and overcome limitations brought on by RA is (in my opinion) about half the battle of living with it.

If you are like me and have RA or are reading in the hopes that you can help a loved one out with their own diagnosis, I truly hope that in each chapter you will find concrete information and new ideas to help you or your loved one live fully, and more pain free.

Before we get started, I want to mention one surprising hurdle I faced, and likely one that you will face, too, because RA is often invisible.

It's surprising to think that my first and most puzzling obstacle would be convincing others that there was something going on with me. But that's exactly what happened. It started shortly after my diagnosis, when my mother-in-law mentioned to me that I didn't "look" like I had anything wrong with me.

How exactly should one look, when they are dealing with something that is battling them from the inside-out?

Although it was a bit of a learning curve for both of us, I have outlined the ways in which I handled this first obstacle in my RA life and set myself on the right path to truly understanding my pain, and furthermore, relaying that information accurately to others.

I've gathered up all this information in a free download just for readers of this book: *"Explaining an Invisible Disability: Helpful Advice on How to Communicate to a Skeptical World When Your Chronic Condition is Invisible."*

To get your copy of this download go to my website www.HelenWardDay.com and click on this image.

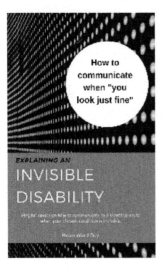

"BUT YOU DON'T LOOK SICK"

I recall a time before my mother-in-law and I were communicating well, when she plopped down a gallon of strawberries and handed me a paring knife and asked me to clean and top them for the lunch she was serving. I did my best with my stiff hands, but she started commenting that I was taking off too much of the top of the strawberry. I was there, head down, blinking away tears of frustration; I was being scolded like a lazy child. All I wanted to do was to melt into the floor and be swallowed up. No-one knew why I was getting emotional. Finally, my husband noticed my distress and took over. That's the problem with RA. Depending on a person's point of view, it can appear as laziness, carelessness, indifference, sloth. And that's not true at all.

Even for the average, healthy person, the winter holidays tend to be a stressful and strenuous time. With cooking, cleaning, preparing for guests, buying and wrapping presents and everything else that holidays throw at us, it's only natural for us to be pretty exhausted. Now, take that feeling, and throw in a chronic illness that saps your everyday energy and move-

ment. RA and the holidays were like a KO punch to any resolve
I had about tackling my illness to live fully. I was just *tired.*

My mother-in-law was not the type to let something go
unseen or unspoken. We had a solid relationship, but she
was always very forthcoming with her thoughts—even when
they were a little insensitive.

She mentioned to me one year that I always "ruined the
holidays." Specifically, she said I made them less enjoyable
because I was always sick, getting sick, just getting over being
sick, and/or dealing with something, even when I didn't look
ill. She went so far as to say she thought it was all in my head
and an avoidance tactic to skip out on family gatherings. She
said I needed counseling.

It was a real bummer to hear that my efforts to put forth my
best were not only *failing*, but that I was bringing other people
down because of an illness that I had no part in asking for. I felt
defeated; what small inkling I had left of wanting to be a part of
the festivities died out pretty fast after her statement.

I reveal all this, not to make her look bad, but to shed light
on what others were probably thinking, even if she was the only
one saying it out loud.

The thing is, RA isn't an ailment that you can point out on a
person. And I realized soon after that to most people, common ailments and illnesses are easily recognizable; that's part of
what makes them *common.*

It takes only a few moments to create a judgement about
someone, even if it's just a person you walked past on the street.
If you see them in a three-piece suit, well-fitted and a very clean
haircut and trimmed beard, you can assume that they are a
person of high wealth, education, and/or class/merit. (Again,
not always the case, but you know what they say about
assumptions.)

The same goes for illnesses. Upon gazing at someone, it's more comfortable and digestible to know immediately

what you are dealing with and what to expect. But
RA doesn't work like that. RA doesn't give you many outward
signs, many red flags to throw up and alert people of your
illnesses. It's mostly invisible.

THE INVISIBLE ILLNESS

Rheumatoid arthritis is often known as one of the "invisible
illnesses," meaning that those who are diagnosed with it don't
usually conform the standards of what many people think "sick"
looks like.

A foot or arm in a cast gets immediate sympathy: others can
feel and understand the pain because they can *see* the pain on
the outside. Cast = injury. But when you're battling with painful
motion, constant aches, and stiff joints, it doesn't come across
the same. Even harder to explain is that RA is a fluctuating
condition. Some days I can do certain tasks with ease.
Other days, I struggle and need help taking the tops off
of strawberries.

Just like with my mother-in-law—who couldn't really
understand the pain that I was going through because it was
internal and fluctuating—you might find yourself dealing with
similar situations over time.

TAKE THE TIME TO EXPLAIN

An approach to dealing with these complications that I found
useful was to first, understand what I was up against fully. I did
this by spending a lot of time reading, researching, and talking
with others who have RA.

When I was able to understand RA better myself, only then I
was able to share that knowledge to others around me. It's easy

to boil it down to as *"I'm just tired"* or *"My hands/wrists/knees/feet are bothering me."* But the more detail you include about what's really going on, the better others are at truly understanding. A phrase I learned that seemed to break through to some people was to describe RA as sometimes having "flu-like symptoms." That's something most people recall vividly.

I think anyone with a chronic illness emphatically does not want to become that person who can only harp on what ails them. I really, really, really do not want to devolve into that stereotype. But it is perfectly fine to take the time to help others realize that it's not just *pain*; RA can cause malaise, fever, memory issues, weight loss and depression. RA can affect more than just the joints—if you're like me, dealing with multiple chronic illness at once, it can complicate or exacerbate others you are already dealing with.

Initially, I found myself struggling with how to approach my mother-in-law, and others, who had misconceptions about RA. I didn't want to come off as angry or irritated that they were misinformed—although, I know some of that lingered some-where underneath the surface—I just wanted them to under-stand. To have empathy. To be patient. I was trying my hardest to live just as I had always done.

I explained not just RA and what it could do, but also what I was currently feeling, what I might feel in the future as it progressed, what medications and treatments I was on and how that effected my day-to-day tasks. It took a while, and multiple conversations and although I felt like I was sharing too much, it really opened the eyes of my mother-in-law and how she un-derstood what I was dealing with.

A good way to open up these conversations, if you're not sure where to start, is to explain the differences between a commonly known illness—osteoarthritis—and RA.

Arthritis is an umbrella term for inflammation of the joints. So, both osteoarthritis and rheumatoid stem from this common problem with the body—and that's about where the similarities end.

Most people will be familiar with osteoarthritis, a degenerative disease caused by the wear and tear on joints. Osteoarthritis is linked to repetitive movements and pressure placed on the joints—during job activities or when performing hobbies—while the underlying cause of RA is unknown. Since RA is an autoimmune disorder, the body recognizes the lining around your joints as a threat—like the system's usual response to a virus or an infection—and attacks it.

Taking the time to go through these two illnesses and explain that both have their own additional symptoms and characteristics is a great start.

It's also important to recognize and accept the differences you'll experience after having these conversations. Most will heed what you say and start to look at you differently—which is not always a bad thing.

I found that after explaining my RA, my close friends and family were more willing to help when they saw me struggling, or pick up my slack, so to speak. It may seem frustrating that others feel it necessary to do so, but it can be a real blessing. Some days you don't have the choice to decline offers of help—you simply *need* it.

I hope at least some of this resonates with you and can help you communicate well with others.

For more tips, check out the free download mentioned in the introduction.

CONNECT WITH OTHERS

Unbeknownst to me before my diagnosis, there were already a lot of factors set in place to build a community I was comfortable around and could relate to. I was able to find nonprofit organizations and support groups dedicated to RA, in addition to talking to others online.

Thankfully, RA has slowly gained a greater awareness because of social media and medical studies. If you post in an online forum, most of the time the ones who relate closest to you—i.e., others diagnosed with RA—are not the only ones who may run across your thread. Medical professionals take these testimonies from RA patients and use them, so don't be afraid of social media as a way to document your process for yourself and others as well.

Additionally, you should encourage those around you who don't seem to really "get it" to do their own research. This might not work for everyone who asks questions, but some may glean a bit more information than what you have the time and energy to provide.

RA has a following on social media using the hashtag #invisibleillnessawareness that tracks others who are going through the same difficulties you are. Additionally, it's a great way to not only express some of your personal frustrations, but to find others and build a community of people you can talk to and rely on if needed.

With this thought in mind, I started working on a Facebook group called Inflammation Connection, dedicated to RA and other inflammatory diseases. If you'd like to join this smallish, private group, (get in on the ground floor, so to speak) we'd love to have you. Go to https://www.facebook.com/groups/inflammationconnection.

Additionally, there are many, many websites to educate you further on RA, or lead some of your family and friends toward their own research—and you can find information for all age groups. Be sure to check out the resources at the end of this book. And if by chance you're reading this in print, and a bunch of URLs really don't help much, there's an email address to

contact and I'll happily send you an email with live links to
save your hands from a lot of picky keyboarding.

The Invisible Disability Project publishes information about
invisible disabilities through their website, which boasts a
section for useful vocabulary and testimonial videos from
others with RA.

The Arthritis Foundation also has their own website which
breaks down the different types of arthritis. This can be supple-
mental to what I mentioned above—as well as provide other
useful information like healthy living tips and statistics on
arthritis cases across the United States.

There are also personal blogs written and updated by those
with RA who are trying to build a better, more informed
community for those with autoimmune disorders. Try looking
at some of these blogs—Carla's Corner, Chronic Eileen, or
Arthritic Chick—if you're interested in reading about a more
personalized experience. If you are like me, sometimes you'll
think, "Yeah. That's exactly what I'm dealing with."

CATALOG WHAT'S MOST IMPORTANT TO FOCUS ON

Addressing situations head-on will allow you to use your time
wisely for other tasks that are important to you. I was able
to educate my mother-in-law, and when we got past
her first misunderstanding of RA, the next time I was over for a
family gathering we were able to focus more on the importance
of why we were all there: for fun and for spending time together. Not grading my ability to wield a paring knife.

The same principles apply to everyday life. I don't fret over
the thought that today I needed a mid-day nap in order to continue with my tasks; instead, I focus on the energy that the nap
fueled me with to finish cleaning the stove and counters in the

kitchen. I focus on the sense that in some way, I have beaten RA for just a moment, even if it's a minute victory.

These small victories come because I have mastered the art of cataloging tasks so I can accomplish the most while expending the least amount of energy. This is a thought that I apply in my everyday life to many different situations. While doing yard work, I tend divide each big task into smaller tasks, or "mini projects."

For example, when pulling weeds, I am putting pressure on parts of my body by bending over, therefore activating different joints and tiring them out. To combat this, I stand up and walk the weeds—in small increments—back and forth across the yard to the compost pile or trash bin in order to walk off some of that pressure. It's little modifications like this that keep me from tiring out before I am able to finish at least some of my tasks. (And bending over is an exercise to help keep you flexible,)

I also have to remind myself the importance of cleaning up in the middle—i.e., during cooking, gardening, or any project. It's helped tremendously with not only pain, but my energy levels as well. I put up tools I don't need any more before taking others out so that I don't have fifty tools or implements to put away when fatigue sets in. And remember, glass half-*full*, not half-empty.

This last tip was especially important in my journey to accommodating the unique challenges that come with an autoimmune disorder. I found that by focusing on what I can do instead of what I can't, I am appreciating my body with all of its limitations. I began to make gradual steps toward a lifestyle that allows me to continue to reach all of my goals—whether they be lifetime ones or everyday tasks.

That brings me to our next topic and one that those with RA know well and most likely struggle with—*energy management.*

RA AND ENERGY MANAGEMENT

I've had RA for more than 15 years now, but oddly enough, people seem to think I am an Energizer Bunny. I am known for getting a lot done. The truth is, I more closely resemble a sloth than a rabbit—just ask my husband. This is because I work really, really hard to eliminate from my life everything that I can so that I can accomplish the important things. I plan and strategize every area of my life to limit my energy expenditure to the bare minimum, so that I have internal resources to enjoy the things that enrich my life.

I don't want to waste my time and life energy doing things that aren't enhancing it. Stay up late to binge watch TV? Not very often. I have to stay well-rested to keep flares at bay. Taking care of dry-clean only clothes that involve multiple trips to the cleaners? Hah. Got rid of them years ago. I wear soft knits these days that stretch to cover whatever shape my body has taken lately.

I am also known for perennially early bedtimes. I probably go to bed immediately after work at least one day a week—that means a marathon 15-hour sleep session. Staying asleep is hard when you're achy. But when you are exhausted, it's both possible and necessary.

My company produces special events—something I love to do—but I have found that for every event I produce, I need to make sure I have at least three consecutive days of non-action for a recovery period.

And then there's the matter of spacing things out, when possible. As I am writing this, I am on the eve of my first free weekend in four weeks. We had a major event one weekend (exciting—our first since Covid-19 shut down events), followed by a staff family Easter Egg Hunt (at my house), followed by a family Easter observation—also at my house. These three-full-weekends crammed together is sub-optimal, to say the least.

So, this weekend I will probably not even leave the porch. I'll start to feel perkier late Saturday—but if I am wise, I will stay put, resting through Monday morning.

Sometimes with RA, I am doing fine and then, without warning, I hit a wall. It's like my batteries just die suddenly. No Energizer Bunnies in sight.

RA is associated with permanently inflamed joints—and that sort of widespread inflammation within the body can lead to fatigue. What others do not realize is that feeling fatigued is much deeper than just a sense of being *tired*.

FATIGUE: A CONSTANT BATTLE

Fatigue has been described by some who experience it as "uncontrollable." It's a feeling of tired so strong that you can't fight it with normal means—sleep, caffeine, general willpower. Why is this?

When dealing with chronic pain, some may find it hard to sleep at night. So, after a long day that has worn you out, you lay down and rest your head on the pillow. In the silence, as you try to drift off into slumber, you realize that you are still aching from the things you tried to accomplish earlier in the day.

That aching leads to a restless night of sleep, tossing and turning and trying to get into a comfortable spot, and then you have to wake up and do the whole thing over again. It's a series of unfortunate events that leads to an extreme amount of *fatigue*.

Fatigue has also been linked to symptoms of depression and anxiety—so not only are we dealing with a disorder that is fighting us from the inside-out, but all of its unwelcome mental and emotional buddies, as well.

When you add physical fatigue to fatigue caused by depression or exacerbated by anxiety, the end result is not only not pretty, it can feel suffocating. One way to fight fatigue in all its forms is to become a superior energy guardian.

USE ENERGY WELL AND WITH INTENTION

So how do we manage it? There are many ways to go about this, but one of the first, and maybe most important things is *recognition*.

Realizing, or coming to terms, with the setbacks that RA introduces into your life is half of the battle. Fatigue, pain, low energy, mood swings, general malaise—are all part of your daily routine now. But what can also be a part of that routine is *maintenance*.

Recognize your energy fluctuations—pay special attention to the lows—and then streamline your processes to use that energy well and with full intention toward your optimal tasks. Don't push yourself too hard, and don't feel guilty for the things that you may have been able to do yesterday that you can't carry out today.

It's okay to pace yourself. It's okay to take a small rest. It's okay to take a big rest—like me, when I take three days of non-activity after a big event just to recover. Do what is best for you and what makes you feel okay about the setbacks that come with RA so you can bounce back better than ever.

If you need a little more help, here a few ways to combat fatigue:

EXERCISE

Exercising regularly can not only combat feelings of fatigue but also other underlying symptoms of RA, as well. Exercise builds the muscles around the joints, making them stronger for the activities that cause wear and tear—such as bending, stretching or lifting. It has also been linked to mood elevation and better sleep. I find that I sleep really well after a combination of exercise and a warm shower.

If you're not sure where to start, you can begin with light stretching after waking up and before going to bed, and then as you get more comfortable you can try out yoga, tai chi, or aerobic exercises like swimming or running/walking a half-marathon—like I did.

Later on, in chapter seven we will talk a little more about exercise. But remember, while it takes energy to get out and exercise, it usually returns to you more than you spent in terms of overall well-being. This is especially true when you find ways to add in daily, gentle exercise.

DIET

In addition to exercise, a well-balanced diet can also positively effect energy levels. Food is fuel. Although in the moment, it may seem like reaching for that fast, greasy (or sweet) choice is the right thing to do, but it's better to eat small, healthy meals throughout the day. Try incorporating foods that are high in fiber, complex carbohydrates, and protein. Additional-

ly, Omega-3 fatty acids—like the ones found in fish and nuts—
are said to combat inflammation within the body, so it can
possibly ease some of the fatigue and swelling associated
with RA.

I would also like to add here that it's okay to reward yourself. Keeping a well-balanced diet at all times with everything
that you may have to deal with during the day is just *hard*. If you
feel like rewarding yourself after a rough day with some ice
cream or cake, do it. (In moderation, of course.) Whatever keeps
you motivated, moving and stress-free is worth keeping within
your daily routines.

A NIGHTLY ROUTINE

As humans, we are generally creatures of habit. I found that
it was easier to fall asleep when I trained myself to do so by
developing a habit and setting up a sleep-supporting environment.

Try doing a few consistent steps every single night before
you go to bed: turn off your electronics, boil a cup of tea, turn
on a lamp, and read a book. It can be a combination of anything
you want, but make sure you do it every night so that your body
associates these things with sleeping. In return, your body will
start to relax itself so that you don't stay awake staring at the
ceiling for a few hours and can gradually combat some of that
fatigue. And when reading at night, make it an actual paper
book, or use a device like a Kindle™ Paperwhite that
does not emit sleep disrupting
light. Don't use your smart phone—they are not great relaxation tools—unless you are listening to soothing music.

Most importantly, a routine will associate your bed with
sleep for your brain. That means, during the day, you have all
the more reason to separate yourself from the thing that you
associate with being sleepy. I've heard that when you don't feel

100%, the last thing you want to do is to give into that feeling. Remember: staying in bed when you awaken can actually exacerbate the malaise you feel, so when you are through resting, it's also important to promptly remove yourself from the bed and don't linger.

And, since I am committed to sharing tips from my own life, here is one that's revamped from your grandmother's day: counting. If you have trouble falling asleep, try counting 150 breaths. (I count one inhalation and one exhalation as one breath.) Counting like this allows my brain to calm down and pushes racing thoughts away, and counting my breaths seems to limit my fidgets and wriggles. If I find myself losing my place, I start with the last number I recall, and go from there, unless my mind has wandered far, far away, in which case I start over. If I make a major toss-and-turn move, I start over. I sometimes seem to doze for an instant only to reawaken—and I just start over. I don't check the clock or obsess about how I really need to get to sleep, I just start counting breaths. I seldom get beyond 75. And this keeps me from getting all worked up over the fact I am not asleep.

Delegate or Delete

To the degree possible, go through your inventory of life tasks and delegate any you can. See if your partner can take over a task and you pick up another one. Can you begin to train your kids to do laundry? I started at age six doing laundry as my "family task." My brother cooked, my sister cleaned, and I, the youngest, did laundry. I am sure I ruined a few things, but my mother decided to teach me, and to this day it is one of my favorite chores, because I happen to be an expert at it.

If something cannot be delegated, does it have to be done at all? Sometimes I find myself thinking of how things "ought" to be and wanting them that way. But when I analyze it, I realize that my idea that this thing "ought" to be done is mere habit, or social norm, and I can eliminate it from my life with little problem. One thing I had to let go of years ago for non-RA-related reasons is a nice, green lawn.

Our trees grew so big they began to shade our once full-sun yard. We fought for years to keep some sort of lawn. I finally gave up and mulched my yard enough to keep the weeds down and began to divide the yard into beds and paths. I added in perennials like monkey grass, aspidistra and fatsia, and finally some ivy is creeping across the ground.

Then as RA began to become an issue, I decided to start "hard gardening" which is basically a term I use to describe putting interesting things that don't die in your yard: fountains, bottle trees, bird feeders, interesting rocks—I love rocks. They don't even need water.

Ask For Help

Despite trying every trick in the book, sometimes I am just tired no matter what I do; I just cannot complete the tasks I've set up for myself. So then, I turn to receiving help from those around me. It's hard to feel like I'm depending on other people, but sometimes, I just need it. My husband is always there to lend a hand with the things I am struggling with.

Living with RA can feel like you've lost control of your life. With an autoimmune disease that fluctuates, you can't predict what your day-to-day life will look like. I like to navigate this feeling by controlling what I can. My husband is especially helpful around the house, but on the days when he is away or I just don't want to ask him for help, I rely on a strategy that has helped me keep housework manageable: *decluttering*.

CLUTTER AND ITS NEGATIVE IMPACT

Decluttering is a form of self-care and once achieved, is a great energy conservator and perhaps even an energy booster when you don't have to deal with all that clutter anymore.

Think about it like this—our homes are our sanctuaries. They are a place of relaxation, a place to kick our feet up, be ourselves, and escape from the noise and commotion of the outside world. When I come into my home, I want it to feel like taking a deep breath of fresh air, like I'm truly able to let go of my worries and stress because I'm within my domain, my sanctuary.

When our homes don't give off that vibe because we have too much "stuff," we end up spending a lot of time doing every-thing *but* relaxing. More stuff = more time cleaning up that stuff, sorting through that stuff, and rebuying that stuff because you thought you were out of it, only to find it hidden behind other stuff.

Not to mention it's pretty anxiety-inducing when your eyes have too much to land on. Relaxation is sometimes determined by the amount of "white space" you have, which is why mini-malists thrive within their wholly uncluttered spaces.

I wrote a book on abundance, and the process of organizing that abundance, called *Organize Your Life*. In the book, I went into detail the number of choices that we are given on a day-to-day basis—everything from choosing dinner from many fast-food restaurants on a given street, to an abundance of material possessions because of self-indulgence—and how it can lead to a life full of chaos.

Acquiring the things you want is not a necessarily bad thing. But, when you acquire too much or have too much to choose from, it becomes an *over*-indulgence and can be an incredibly negative force within your life. Decluttering is a method of getting rid of some of that over-indulgence that I mention within the book.

Decluttering your home can lead to a sense of mindfulness and inner peace. Instead of wasting your time—and more importantly, *your energy*—on repeated cleaning, shuffling and reorganizing, having less of everything can be the first step.

However, having less has always been compared to living simply, and "simple" is a word that has a lot of unnecessary negative connotations behind it. We have turned it into a state of being that means unimportant, uncreative, unworthy of really, *anything*. If a dish on Master Chef is considered *too simple*, the contestant is in deep trouble with the judges.

But here, living a life of simplicity while dealing with an autoimmune disorder is one that should be welcomed. Leading a simple lifestyle is not one that comes naturally to a lot of us— simplicity is acquired over time with many, many choices that we have to continue to make.

With RA, it's important that we understand what helps and what hinders us—and taking a few moments to get rid of what I don't need has always benefited me greatly. There's a sense of renewed freedom that comes with throwing things out. I find myself dreading the time I'll spend doing so when it comes to spring cleaning, but once I get myself settled in front of a space with a black trash bag handy, it's like a different side of me comes out.

And another thing, it just feels good to gather up and donate all of those shoes that no longer fit my ever-evolving feet. I feel downright guilty when I see the waste represented by shoes that only fit a week or so before some new nodules sprang from my feet. Getting them to a place where they might be useful relieves the stress I give myself for being "wasteful."

DECLUTTER EVERYWHERE

Decluttering doesn't have to be limited to one area of your home, either. You can declutter your car, the bathroom counter, your Tupperware™ drawer or any contained chaotic space.

Personally, my workspace within my house is a place that must be decluttered at all times. Although I keep it that way for a clear, focused mind rather than relaxation—because working doesn't always equal a state of relaxation—it helps me function better on both sides of the spectrum. I like to have my papers filed, my notebooks stacked and underneath my riser, my pens capped and replaced in my desk caddy, and the surfaces wiped down from where I may have spilled a drop or two of Diet Coke before I can actually sit down and write a single word of an email, article or chapter.

Take the time to let your eyes land on the parts of your house that stress you out the most—is it sorting the stack of catalogs beside your coffee table? Is it the DVD collection underneath the TV? Is it folding and hanging up clothes after a wash day?

There's a way to declutter a lot of these things just by getting rid of some of what you don't need. Throw away old magazines. Perhaps invest in a binder where you can keep all of your DVD's and throw out the cases that get so mixed up when you pick out a movie. Minimize the number of sleep T-shirts or pants you have so you don't have that many to fold and put away in a drawer already crammed full.

It's also important to note here that clutter doesn't always include the physical things that you can put your hands on. You can declutter your calendar, your phone apps, or your computer desktop—really, anything that affects you look at on day-to-day basis.

I know that when I have a lot of apps on my phone with notifications turned on, I'm always looking at those little red boxes with numbers in them and it gives me a sense of dread. Another email, another notification of a great sale, another reminder to do this or that. I have learned that it's okay to turn off notifications for anything that I don't need, therefore, keeping my phone in a better state where it's more visually pleasing to scroll through.

Your calendar is also a good place to look at decluttering. When I have too many things I'm trying to remember, I tend to write it all down: deadlines, bills due, personal reminders, appointments, grocery lists, etc. It seems like a great way to keep track of everything—and, don't get me wrong, it is—but sometimes when I look down at that calendar at the beginning of the week, I feel like my head is spinning.

An easy way to combat this feeling is to one, keep your calendar in a visible location. That way, if there are important reminders, you will see them even when you're not looking for them. Then, keep track of only the things that are at the forefront of your days—whether that be reminders to pick up prescriptions, important due dates, or a loved one's birthday. By decluttering your calendar of unnecessary notes, you free up space not only on the page but in your mind as well.

DEVELOPING DECLUTTERING HABITS

It helps to think of decluttering not as deprivation by throwing your things away, but as a method of cleansing for your mental and physical well-being. Think of it as a daily process of realizing when you need to organize different parts of your life and take the time to do it while you're thinking about it. With RA, it's always important to compartmentalize the things that we need to do and not overwhelm ourselves with a long list of important tasks that we know we can't carry out quickly and efficiently within a day's time.

With limited energy, you may find yourself feeling defeated

when you can't finish a task. Know that it's okay to put things on pause. This is a mindset I've had to adapt to—I used to refuse to stop a task until I'd completed it, which left me burned out and overexerted, which I paid for later. Now, I realize when I need a break, and I take it. I put the thing I'm working on down "just for now," and make a note to come back to it later when I've recharged.

To combat fatigue while decluttering, give yourself small tasks to start with—such as, reorganizing the top drawer of the bathroom vanity cabinet. Once you do that, if you still feel up to it and have the time, maybe your makeup drawer or bag. Go from task to task and give yourself breaks in between. Don't make the mistake of tackling a big thing—like an entire linen closet—only to run out of energy about the time you've pulled everything out and created an utter disaster in your hallway. Start small: one shelf at a time, or just the sheets, then later, the towels.

Again, you may be the type of person who can deal with clutter and it doesn't make you stressed, anxious or tired. Decluttering may not be for you. There are those of us who love the abundance and thrive within it. That's okay, too. But, if you find yourself in the situations mentioned above, try organizing some of the messier places within your life and see if you can tell the difference afterwards.

In the next section I'll go more in depth on how to declutter from room to room, as well as hacks and tips for shortcuts to cleaning and keeping organized.

HOME AND GARDEN

*I*n addition to decluttering, which can help tremendously with time and energy, it's great to know a few other tips and tricks while going room to room in your house that can speed up the cleaning process.

One thing I've learned is not everything can be done in a day. The house is just too big and there are too many things to tackle to try and do it in one day. I may have been able to do a lot more before RA, but I can't do it now. It can be frustrating at times when I want to go ahead and get it all done so I can sit down and relax. But beating myself up for not being diligent enough with housework doesn't help. I've decided it's not the end of the world if I only vacuum my stairs twice a year.

DON'T MULTI-TASK

As a modern society, we are usually proud to be multi-taskers—it's become one of the skills that prospective employers ask you about. But multi-tasking is sometimes little more than being a "self-interrupter." When you engage in a task, it takes you anywhere from a few seconds, in the case of a simple, mainly manual task, to up to 20 minutes for a complex task that requires concentration, for you to fully engage and be productive. Time spent reengaging over and over it time wasted.

Anyone can put in a load of laundry while paying the bills online. I am not arguing that. But if you are talking to your kids after school, watching the news, paying bills and heating up something for dinner, none of those tasks is getting your full attention.

Multi-taskers often take longer to get things done, and they are more likely to make errors. Because of the frequent changes in thoughts and levels of concentration, it takes a lot more energy to get things done. It's stressful to multi-task.

When you are working around your house, unless there are clearly "background tasks" like running the dishwasher while you vacuum, try to do one major thing at a time. For example, if you need to declutter, organize and then clean an area, first declutter. Then reorganize. And only after that, clean.

HONE YOUR DEFENSES

I have really had to up my defense when it comes to housekeeping. Offense is when you are actively cleaning up, doing necessary chores. But defense is when you are doing things that minimize or eliminate future housework.

A good defense helps you keep chores to a minimum.

Defense might be using paper plates for quick breakfasts.

Defense is rinsing dirty pots and pans before stuff hardens.

Honestly, defense can be having pups in the kitchen, clearing up bits on the floor as you cook.

Defense is getting really good floor mats in the entry way, or becoming a "no shoes" household.

Defense is doing projects and chores in small phases, so you can stop mid-way through without having a semi-disaster on hand. Let me give you an example of this:

Say you are preparing twenty treat bags for a party. You know you want to have them nicely filled, then closed with a ribbon, decorated with flowers, and then personalized with handmade gift tags.

Do this by first filling all the bags. Then close all twenty with the ribbon. If time and energy permit, decorate with flowers. If you're running out of either time or energy, perhaps skip to the name tag, and stop there. If you are still going strong and have the time, then add flowers to all twenty. The point is, if you'd had to stop at any step, you'd still have had twenty ready-to-go, albeit plainer, gift bags. If you had done the first five bags with treats, ribbon, flowers and custom name tags, you'd be forced to do all twenty to that state of completion. Make sense? I try to do most things this way.

A favorite defense of mine is to tidy up as I do things, so I won't have a huge project after I finish my project.

Another defensive technique that is probably specific to me is to break my habit of leaving drawers open about three inches. I have no idea why I do this, but I can assure you, having a drawer open three inches in the kitchen almost guarantees I am going to spill something that runs into the drawer, making a huge mess. Defense is simply closing drawers before disaster strikes.

PLAN AHEAD

I've found that when I am preparing for an event—say, the family is coming over for dinner on Saturday night—I make a plan a few days before it to tackle each room. I space it out over the week so that I can really focus on what needs to be done without exhausting myself. Remember, prioritizing is a big part of the process here. Put the most important things first, and get rid of anything that doesn't absolutely need to be done. If I have the time and energy I can tackle some lower priorities later.

Additionally, even when I don't have a big event coming up, I find that cleaning small amounts here and there is helpful throughout the week. It's always a good idea to tackle smaller jobs when I have a spare moment, like wiping down counters in the kitchen or emptying the trash cans in the bathroom when they're full.

Each room has its own unique challenges to keeping it neat and tidy, so we'll start with the living room—which is always important to keep clean because it's where guests will convene and is also where I spend most of my time when I'm in the house.

LIVING ROOM OR DEN

Vacuuming

One of the most daunting chores in my household is vacuuming: lugging that big machine everywhere and then pushing it across all the floors in my house was a huge task even before my RA hit. I have invested in a smaller, more lightweight, cordless vacuum that has really been all the difference in conserving my energy. Mine is the Bissel™ Featherweight Cordless Stick™, but there are plenty others that will do the trick just as well. I like the ones that have the "hammerhead shark" shaped intake, that rests on the floor when you vacuum. That eases the strain I feel when I must carry the entire weight of the battery pack in one hand.

In more recent years, I've gone even further with upgrading my cleaning tools and invested in a Roomba™ knock-off. It's a very small little cleaning robot that roams around my house and picks up and debris, crumbs, or dust lying about while I busy myself with other things. It's amazing. Although some can be on the pricier side, there are also some cheaper options out there, so shop around.

DUSTING

I like to use a dryer sheet for dusting. It's a great way to use the products you might already have in a different way—especially great when they're cheap and come in a large quantity—and keeps me from accumulating too many tools in the house. You can use them on TV screens, blinds, entertainment systems, and more.

On days when my hands are less nimble, I like to use Swiffer™dusters. They are lightweight and kind of fun to use. (Probably thanks to great marketing.)

Otherwise, if you like an old-fashioned ostrich feather duster, make sure it's one with an extendable and retractable handle in order to reach all of the places needed. Both vacuuming and dusting need to be done in small increments—only do what you can and listen to your body when it tells you to take a break. These can be draining tasks, but only if you let them be.

One last note about dusting—play good defense and keep knick-knacks to a minimum. And if you do have beloved items on display, make sure they are heavy enough that you can dust around them without having to pick each one up.

I have a collection of ceramic dog figures I have collected over the years, and I finally invested in a glass-fronted display case to avoid the need to dust around them.

FURNITURE

This may seem like a no-brainer to some, but sometimes we just don't have our furniture and other pieces aligned in a way that is making the most use out of a space. Equally, furni-

ture positioning poses a lot of influence in how we navigate a
space. It's especially important to consider this when you
make use of a walker or cane during your day-to-day activity.
If you find yourself struggling with this, you can declutter
your living area by getting rid of pieces of furniture that
you don't need.

Over the years we have acquired from relatives two end
tables, but no matter how I rearranged the room with my husband, I couldn't figure out how to make it so the end
table wasn't in the way. In the end, I wound up finding only one
end table useful, and I put the other in a bedroom, where it now
serves as a very nice nightstand.

It's easy to accumulate too much furniture after years and
years of living in one place, so it may be time to part with some
of those things to make maneuvering the space a bit easier for
not only you and your family, but your guests as well.

DINING ROOM AND KITCHEN

There are tons and tons and tons of hacks for the kitchen—
almost too many to decide which ones are most important. I
will try to list some here that address actual cleaning and maintenance. In the next chapter I will go further into detail
about cooking in the kitchen and doing laundry.

DECLUTTER FIRST

Start your kitchen cleaning by decluttering wherever possible. Toss out ancient spices that you can't recall ever using, expired canned foods, frozen objects in zipper bags in the freezer
with no dates and no labels. Bit by bit, declutter one small area
at a time. The more you declutter the less you have to clean. If
you don't know where to start, try starting with a junk draw-

er. How many little boxes of partially melted birthday candles do you really need to keep on hand?

DEEP CLEANING

Here, I make the most of my cleaning products, so they do more of the work than I do. If you have a tile backsplash in your kitchen, the same Scrubbing Bubbles spray that would normally be for the bathroom can be used. I like to spray and let it soak—again, it does me a favor by lifting some of the grime so that I don't have to scrub as hard—and then I follow up with my mop or Swiffer. By using the same product for two different jobs, you can also consider this a method of decluttering.

Any spray cleaner should be left on at least three minutes to let it get its work done. Wiping any sooner is more work for you and uses more product when you have to reapply. If you need a gentle scraper for dried on gunk on your counter or stove top or floor, soak it with cleanser and then scrape with an expired credit card. (Or stiff plastic spatula.)

When cleaning your oven, don't get impatient. If the instructions say wait overnight, wait overnight. I have discovered that if things aren't clean the first go-round, it's easier to wipe everything out and run the cycle again—chemical or self-cleaning—both are easier on the back and hands if you apply time rather than brute force scrubbing.

I am also a huge fan of Clorox Wipes. They were hard to find during the pandemic, so I guarded my supply carefully. But in more abundant times, they make quick work of "fresh" messes and sanitize while tidying up.

DISHES, POTS AND PANS

Loading the dishwasher is yet another hurdle to overcome in the kitchen, so a lot of times I choose to put away the good china and use paper plates. Although it's not the most appealing to the eyes, and my mother-in-law would highly disagree with my thought process behind this, it really does wonders for cleaning up. There are no dishes to rinse and put on the rack, there is nothing to put away after washing—it's just use and dispose. Now, don't get me wrong: I do reach for my wedding china when there are bigger plans. But for those nights during the week when it's just a simple dinner for me and my husband, paper plates are my go-to.

I like to use a soap-dispensing brush for pots and pans. I fill it up once and I don't have to keep dish soap on my countertop —which keeps me from having more to move around and clean later. Additionally, cleaning the pots I use quickly keeps the grease and grime from sticking/hardening. If I did it later, I would spend more time scrubbing at things that got stuck to the bottom and sides, so my soap-dispensing brush is the most useful when I act quickly.

Another hack for cleaning pots and pans is to fill them up after you're through using them—almost as if you're going to let them "soak" in the sink—but put them back on the stove and let them heat up. The heat will activate the soap inside and loosen up some of those stuck-on food particles, making it easier to clean. Just wait until it cools down again to actually take your sponge to it, of course. Oh—and if you're like me, and might forget your simmering "self-cleaning" pot, set a timer. That has saved me more times than I like to admit.

And a final tip: for pots and pans, if you are going to soak them in the sink, fill them to the brim. In our house, unless there has been a cooking accident, the sides of the pots are usually harder to clean than the bottom—which has generally been kept moist during the cooking process while the sides of the pot open to air.

STORAGE

In order to declutter the kitchen cabinets and countertops, I make use of one: a spice rack, and two: organization tools within my pantry. I used to be the type of person that just threw something behind a closed door in my kitchen and then worried about it only later when I reopened that door and something came crashing out. Now, I have realized the importance of organization. Invest in a labeled spice rack, organize your pantry with storage bins, and get that pot and pan collection minimized and in order. It will save you a ton of time later—not only when you're looking for something, but when it's time to put everything away after you've used them.

The refrigerator is another place I tend to neglect when it comes to storage or cleaning. I am always packing away yummy leftovers from dinner and placing them in the back of the fridge, only to forget about them. Then, I open the door one day and realize something has gone bad because of an uninvited stench that is wafting out—and low and behold, there it is. Last week's lasagna, tucked away in the back of my fridge in a Tupperware bowl I have been looking for the last few days.

So, don't be like me. Clean out your refrigerator and freezer regularly. Even a simple wipe-down of the shelves and walls every once in a while, is helpful. By doing so, you will be saving yourself time and money because you'll constantly be taking notice of the inventory you have for the next time you go to grocery store. The same goes for your pantry—watch those expiration dates.

There are also many products for the kitchen that can help with accessibility. If you are able to do a bit of remodeling to your home, there are wall shelves that can be placed inside of cabinets so that you are able to pull the rack up and out for easier access. You can also place items that you use often within sliding drawers, if possible. Tip: Remember: bring the objects you need to you, don't reach for them. Additionally, placing them within eye-level will keep you from stooping or stretching.

One kitchen accessory that I stumbled upon a few years back was a free-standing, wrought iron pot stand. It keeps all our pots in sight, neatly arranged from largest (and heaviest) at the bottom to the smaller ones at the top. No bending, except for the bottom shelf, where we keep the cast-iron Dutch oven. It also makes selecting a pot easy, as all your choices are in plain sight. This three-legged rack even manages to organize my husband's collection of large stock pots for his bulk cooking. We liked this thing so much that when we redid our kitchen, we made sure there was still room for it.

Don't Specialize Too Much

By this I mean to keep your kitchen as open and functional as possible, consider limiting your collection of highly specific counter-top appliances if you have limited counter space. Crock pot, air fryer, bread machine (remember those?), toaster, toaster-oven, food steamer, food processor, stand mixer, blender, juicer, indoor electric grill, yogurt-maker, coffee apparatus, instant pot, rice steamer—it is amazing the plethora of supposedly time- or work-saving devices you can add to your arsenal in the kitchen. But unless you are going to use an appliance multiple times per week, consider using a more generic alternative instead.

We once had a countertop electric food steamer. It was handy. But it did the exact same thing as a pot with a few ounces of water in the bottom. And it took up space. Crumbs found their way underneath it, and it had a half dozen parts and accessories. And now it is gone. And we are back to our classic pots that work just fine.

Don't give in to the latest cooking gadget fad without knowing how easy is it to use, how hard is it to clean, and where it will live when not in use. Ask yourself how many times you will use it after the first 30 days. And does it require special accessories or food items (K Cups®) to use it?

If you find a time or energy saving tool that makes your life easier, great. Just don't buy every one that hits the market without making sure you have room in your kitchen for it.

BATHROOM

Bathrooms are a tricky place—not just for cleaning, but also maneuvering in the space physically. The bath is the smallest space in the house that we frequent multiple times each day, which makes it prone to getting dirty and needing a little extra TLC and thought behind our decision-making.

For me, I have found that the worst time of my day for me RA-wise is the time of day I spend the most time in the bathroom—first thing in the morning. When I get up my feet are practically rigid, and my ankles don't bend. So, I wind up doing a stiff-legged shuffle into a room created to offer slip and fall hazards. That means I need to spend extra effort to keep it neat, clean and clutter free.

BATHTUB, TOILET, AND FLOORS

The tub in my house was always a place where I wanted to throw up the white flag and call it a day. It required a lot of bending, a lot of vigorous scrubbing, and unfortunately, put a lot of pressure on my knees when I had to squat/sit to reach all the nooks and crannies. Nowadays, I find it easier to use products that I can spray and let sit, so that it soaks off all the grime and I have less scrubbing to do when it comes to soap scum and water stains. Use a small folding stool handy so that you can sit and reach—rather than bending or squatting—and don't forget to take breaks.

For the toilet, I have invested in a few things that make the cleaning process a bit easier. In line with my soaking saves

energy philosophy, I use those bleach tablets you put in your
toilet tank. I've also found you can buy long-handled toilet
brushes. MATCC Shower Scrubber™ works fine on toilet
bowls. OXO Good Grips™ has an extendable brush and scrubber. And for quick touch up, there are Clorox™ Toilet Wands
with disposable wand heads.

Scrubbing Bubbles™ are my friend for both bathtub and
toilet.

For floors, I like to turn my little robot vacuum cleaner loose
(trapping him in there to do a thorough job). Then I go over
the floor with a Swiffer™ Wet Mop.

I have seen ads for electric or battery-operated scrubbing
spinners to assist in bathroom cleanup, but I hate to add
another tool when what I am doing works so far. Maybe later, if
hand strength becomes a bigger issue, I might consider one.

Spray bottles and spray cans are always problematic for
me. It's hard to both grip and press down or grip and squeeze
because they can be so slippery. Rubber bands around the
bottles help a lot, even if my hands get wet. If possible, I like to
hold the item in the store to see if my small hands fit
around it.

If damp tools become too slippery or difficult to manage see
about getting some foam grip tools. I found a pack of six, with
two each of three different diameters. You can cut off just as
much as you need, so you get multiple uses from each tube.
They can fit over everything from brush handles to tooth-
brushes.

Other accessibility items you might want to consider are
things that make your bathroom easier for you to use. As
mentioned above, foam grips can make a toothbrush easier to
use. You can put such a grip on a disposable razor, too, and
simply move it to the new one each time you change.

Pump shampoos and conditioners help with dispensing
product. And if you ever gave your dad some, don't forget "soap

on a rope." They make many fine soaps available this way, and the ropes keep them under control.

If you use a shower bench or seat, consider getting a showerhead to help eliminate twisting and turning.

And don't forget those tacky (literally) little stickers for slippery surfaces. They may be something you used as a child, but anything to help you keep your footing is worth it.

Bathroom Accessibility Aids

According to the CDC (The Centers for Disease Control & Prevention), the bathroom is the most dangerous room in your house. This means that for people with limited mobility, balance issues, and other functional disabilities, investing in appropriate accessibility aids in the bathroom is critical.

I hate to say this out loud, but if you go online and search for "bathroom aids for the elderly" you will hit the jackpot on products designed to make your life easier. And I know, it's hard to say, "I'm going to set my bathroom up like I am an elderly person." But studies have shown that seniors who equip their homes with safety features and accessibility aids remain in their homes longer than those who do not make accommodations to their stage in life.

So, while I've mentioned a few tools already, I want to encourage you to do an honest assessment of how you function in your bathroom and then research tools that will help you avoid the pitfalls.

There are grab bars, elevated toilet risers, frames to go around your toilet to help you lift yourself up, bath seats that let you sit down outside of your tub and slide yourself over.

There are slip resistant mats, padding that can be placed on sharp edges, and night lights to help you see where you are going without blinding yourself with a blast of light late at night.

My personal issues are extreme stiffness in the mornings,

meaning I don't even attempt to step in my tub. We are fortu-
nate to have a "near" walk-in shower. Whoever decided to leave
a four-inch threshold to step over, however, needs a good
talking to.

When staying in hotels with step in tub-shower combos, I
am always very wary. In addition to stiffness, I find myself with
balance issues. If I had to use a step-in tub all the time, I'd invest
in one of those assist railings that slip firmly over the side, and
let you balance by holding firm to the support until you are
secure in your footing.

If you rent, you may be able to get your landlord to install
grab bars. But if that is not an option, there are strong suction
cup versions.

Some of these tools need to be installed professionally. If
you can't locate someone who can help you, consider calling
your local council on aging to see if they have any recommen-
dations.

STORAGE

Decluttering comes back into play here. I know it's very
easy to stack everything up on your counter and have it accessible during the week. But when you go to clean, you have
to take all of it off, and then put it back up there in a neater
way. So, bathroom storage is a *must*. But, as we have
discussed earlier—the important first step is to clear out all the
stuff you don't need, don't use or is expired. That will go a long
way toward making your bathroom easier to deal with. And
if you're someone who likes to experiment with various
personal care products, finish the old one first, or
toss what's left of it.

Keeping your counter clean and uncluttered makes it easier
to wipe down quickly, saving you time and energy in the long
run. Use storage bins or wall mounted holders to keep hair dry-
ers/wands/straighteners and their cords tucked away nicely.

You can also invest in drawer organizers if you have a lot of small makeup items or jewelry. Items that tend to come in big packs—i.e., cotton swabs or pads—can be placed in clear, reusable containers to keep them tidy and visible.One hack I learned from going on cruises—which have microscopic bathrooms—is to hang a clear plastic shoe holder over the door. There are lots of pockets and I can see everything without stooping to open drawers. At first, I thought it might look strange to use one at home, but I even get compliments on it.

It's also important to remember to keep your cleaning supplies nearby. If you have them handy, it's easier to wipe things down periodically instead of making a separate trip into another room to get them. Keep disinfectant wipes under the counter for easy surface cleaning, place your shower cleaner somewhere near the shower, and your toilet brush nearby in the corner.

If I must go to a different room to get something, I'll get distracted while on my way, check the mail, eat lunch, walk the dogs, and then weed a flowerbed, only to get back to the bathroom later and wonder why I left it half-cleaned.

BEDROOM

If you've ever watched a fitness YouTuber's "day in my life," you know that most of them start off every day with making their bed. It's a simple task that seems unimportant—considering you leave your bed for most of the day and then don't return to it until nighttime—but it really makes a difference when you have limited energy and mobility. Take the time after getting out of bed to flip back your sheets and covers and make them look nice. I promise that it won't only save you time and energy later, but it will make you feel more productive throughout the day to see that your bed is made.

Just like there are many tools available to assist in the bathroom, there are specific tools for bedrooms.

Bed risers can be a convenient tool that make getting in and out of bed a little bit easier if you find yourself struggling with that somedays. Just like with a car that's too low, getting in and out of your bed when it's very close to the floor can also put unnecessary strain on your joints, so raise it up a little.

Now, raising your bed up may make you more tempted to store things underneath it because of the provided space. This is a no-go. It will only make it easier to turn it into a place full of clutter, and make it harder to retrieve those things because of the inconvenience of having it on the floor and underneath something. It's also a tripping hazard if a shoe or storage bin happens to be sticking out, which is no good for anyone. Place items where you can easily access them; if shoes are a big problem for you, get a clear, over-the-door organizer. If books or knickknacks are a problem, try using more shelving, but make sure to keep it neat and tidy.

When it comes to beds, generally the most taxing part is changing the sheets. I have found myself literally out of breath with wrangling the mattress to get the bottom sheet on tightly. One help I have discovered is a nifty thing called (unimaginatively) Bed Made EZ Bed Maker Kit. That's a long name for a simple set of plastic wedges you push under the corners of your mattress to give you space to get the fitted sheets in place. They work.

And while we are talking about sheets, moving around in the bed, under sheets and covers, is sometimes difficult. I accidentally stumbled upon a great helper in maneuvering in and out of and around the bed: satin pajamas.

I never use flannel pajamas anymore, nor those nice, soft knit sheets. They would stick to me like Velcro™. I use plain cotton. When wearing satin pajamas, the plain cotton sheets, no matter what their thread count, make an excellent surface to slip and slide all over. I no longer find myself trapped in twisted sheets wrapped around my legs. My legs are my stiffest limbs and any ease I can give them is great. Just be careful when sitting up on the side of the bed. If your feet aren't anchored you can slip and slide right off the bed.

There are standing aids which slide between mattress and box spring and brace against the floor—creating a strong anchor to assist you in sitting up and then standing.

If your feet are tender and achy, there are sheet risers that lift the bedding off of your feet. They come in a foam block style, that you put under the top sheet at the end of the bed. Other styles (sometimes called blanket lifters) tuck into the seam between mattress and box spring at the foot of the bed and are more stationary. Some even come with clamps that can be used to keep your sheets and blankets in place.

After a review of your bedroom, research "bedroom aids for the elderly" to find all sorts of tools and gadgets that might be helpful for you.

One last tip: now that we've all got so many electronic devices in our lives (and on our nightstands), make sure you keep your chargers and cords up and out of the way, so you are not creating additional trip hazards.

GARAGE

My best advice for garage hacks is to make sure you have the best access to the things you need most often. Don't put your everyday items up high on shelves or risers if you cannot reach them without strain or stretch. Save the out-of-the-way storage locations for things you only need a few times (or once) a year. The things you use over and over should be kept in easy reach, generally from chest to knee level.

When storing boxes, label their contents on all sides—I even do the top. After I started doing this, I found it saved me from being in the hot (or chilly) garage, opening box after box, looking for something specific. Over time, I have gotten quite detailed in my content descriptions.

Another thing I have learned from my years as an event planner is to put things away in condition to use them again right out of the box. At the end of an event, when everyone is exhausted, it's easy to toss something in a box, knowing it's a mess. You tell yourself that you'll get it back out before you need it again and set it to rights, but then you don't. And months later, when you pull it out again you see that it requires repair, sorting, cleaning or parts and supplies that you don't have time to deal with. Put things away properly now, even if it takes longer, and you'll be much happier in the long run.

Make it a point to store like things together: gardening stuff all together, automotive stuff together, household tools organized and together.

One last thing about storing things in the garage—do the last fifteen seconds of any "putting-away" task. Don't get all the way out to the garage to put away a cordless drill, and then put it on top of a bin of kids' toys, "just for now." That's a disaster in the making. It will be covered with six other "just-for-nows" before long, and the next time you need it, you'll spend half an hour locating it. Go ahead and put it completely away. All the way down to and including the accessories neatly in the box. You'll thank yourself later.

Invest in a short, sturdy, but lightweight step ladder. I have one that is aluminum that has three wide steps that can accommodate my whole foot, so my body weight is not concentrated on one area. It also has a wide platform for the top step. Then, the handle I use to move it around doubles as a guard rail at the top. So, with even the firm footing it provides, there is a nice grab bar built in. It's light and folds to less than three inches deep—so it fits just about anywhere. Big box stores carry these.

Buy one in person to make sure you get the. Lightest one that will do the trick.

If you find yourself standing in the garage in one place for long periods of time, invest in an anti-fatigue mat. Not only are these much easier on your feet, they also help insulate your feet from the cold concrete floors in winter.

If you can make your garage door motorized, do so to keep yourself from pulling it opened and closed and putting more strain on yourself physically.

Garages are known as the second-most likely place in your home to have excess clutter—the first being the attic—so take a few moments to make sure you have your things organized, put away, and labeled. Also, like the other rooms of the house that you may have decluttered already: get rid of anything you don't need. Some homeowners like to use the garage as a place to park their cars. (Yeah. Unimaginative.)

YARD AND GARDEN

One of my favorite places at my home is my garden. It's a hobby that started off small and blossomed into a safe, relaxing place that I find myself coming back to time and time again. I love getting lost in repotting plants, taking care of something, and watching it grow, and the absolute joy of eating something that is home grown. Sometimes my cherry tomatoes don't even make it inside the house because they are just so delicious.

Before RA I used to occasionally get up as early as 4:00 am (I know, crazy) to get in a good yard session before getting to work by eight. Turning over a compost pile by streetlight is weird, but that's how much pleasure I got from being in my yard. Some people work out before work—I'd work in my garden.

But over the years, as my RA has progressed, I am learning that our double lot—which was a selling point when we bought the house—sometimes feels more like a curse now.

I still garden. But I've transitioned from labor intensive plants and annuals to low-maintenance perennials. Monkey grass is now my friend. I do keep a few smaller beds to plant in, so I get that "up-to your-elbows-in-dirt" feeling, but now I have more container plants. I have also started dabbling in Bonsai, which I find relaxing. It's more labor-intense than you think, but we're talking minutes each day, not hours. I also have a hydroponic growing system in the window of the kitchen. If we can't have home grown tomatoes and beans and squash year-round, at least we have fresh herbs. And for a super-low maintenance window garden, I keep a variety of air plants that I mist daily.

Gardening has been proven to help mind, body and spirit. It can lower stress and alleviate depression. But, when our disabilities get in the way of that, how do we continue to incorporate the things that we love? I'll start with the smallest change that has helped me tremendously with my garden: *tools.*

TOOLS

You've probably seen or used those grabber tools that allow you to get things from overhead in your home. Did you know there are also gardening grabber tools? They can save you lots of bending over. I've used one in my moss-covered Fairy Garden to pick up the giant oak leaves that fall on the delicate moss. So easy.

If you find yourself reaching and bending a lot when tending to your garden, invest in something that will bring the items to you; there are also extendable handle gardening tools. Most have been manufactured to be lightweight and strong with comfortable grips for your hands. You can use these grabber tools on leaves, grass trimmings, or garden foliage.

In addition, there are also elevated planter bed kits that can be used to ease accessibility concerns. Raised beds come in a variety of styles, shapes and sizes, and can also be customized to have watering systems, shelters and pest barriers. Any handyman can build raised beds for you.

A rolling garden chair or stool can help you navigate your garden rows, especially if they are narrow, and will reduce the amount of mobility needed to reach all of your plants. Pair this with a rolling cart that carries all of your tools —or a gardening belt, if you can find one that is lightweight and comfortable—and you've cut your movement by half. At one point I carried a five-gallon bucket with a canvas pouch wrap on it to hold tools. But now anything I do lop-sided, or with one side of my body, tends to give me problems. I focus on solutions that roll.

And while we're talking tools, get either a kneeling bench, which is a low padded bench with sturdy arms to lift yourself up with—or, my favorite, a sit-upon plastic gardening cart. They even open up to carry small tools and gloves, and then you pull it by the handle back to the garage when you are finished. I've mastered the side-scootch, where you use your feet to propel yourself sideways without getting up. These are super handy for doing anything you need to squat to do.

The balls of my feet simply won't flex far enough to let me squat anymore—so I've even brought one of these carts into the house to use when cleaning out low drawers, or sorting the bottom of a closet, or cleaning the tub. And they make base-boards a breeze.

Another gardening hack is to use those endless Amazon shipping boxes as weed receptacles. Bags flop and squash, and even blow away. Your cardboard box just sits there, open, waiting for you to toss in the next weed. Dealing with weeds is much easier when you are not struggling with a flimsy bag. I then place the box at the curb on trash day. Easy.

Growing From Seed

Rather than replanting plants you purchase in those plastic six and eight packs, it may save you some energy to grow your fruits, vegetables, or flowers from seed right in the bed. The only thing you have to do is keep them watered following germination and maybe watch for voracious squirrels. (Cayenne pepper helps me with that, I buy it from Dollar Tree™.). Prepare yourself for some unsuccessful tries—but it is easier, especially if you have those raised planter beds that I mentioned before. Planting starter plants in those plastic packs you get at the gardening store require a lot more kneeling, bending and digging. And dealing with getting the plants out of their plastic housing is very difficult for me to do without mangling the plant or its roots because of my balky fingers—made even more clumsy when wearing garden gloves.

Planting Annuals and Other Starter Plants

If growing from seed isn't your forte—and it wasn't mine for many years—I do have a shortcut for planting those plastic six-packs that spring plants come in. Get a cheap, rechargeable drill and an auger, which looks like a giant screw. When I add to my annual monkey grass expansion project, I buy flats (36 plants) of monkey grass and use the auger on the drill to make all the holes. Just make sure the drill you buy has enough power for the auger you select. It still requires some bending and stooping (less if using a garden seat or cart), but I can plant a flat of monkey grass in less than an hour this way.

· · ·

WATERING

It's an essential—and sometimes, difficult—task to complete depending on the size and depth of your garden. With watering, it's important to invest in tools that extend your reach, so you are covering wide areas without sapping your energy. So, when you are choosing the space for your garden, something to consider is how close it is to a source of water; you don't want to put it on a part of your yard where the hose is on the complete opposite side.

For better reach, try a watering wand that is attachable to a hose end. You can also consider a setting up a sprinkling system or a hose attachment with different nozzles that will help your plants depending on what they need—while some plants get beaten down by hard streams, and some may need just a light misting, some may really need a good soaking. To the degree you can set up a system at the beginning of the season and leave it in place, the less energy you will spend. I only have one spigot in my yard and was constantly having to disconnect and reconnect the sprinkler hose and the watering wand. I found a splitter in the hardware store and bought another hose. Now I just twist the lever on the splitter and choose which hose I want to use, the one with a sprinkler or the one with the watering wand. And I can leave the sprinkler hose in place all summer.

When shopping for water wands or hose nozzles, look for ones that can be locked into position. That way you don't have to squeeze the lever the entire time you are watering.

One final note: more plants die from over watering than under watering—especially container plants.

WEEDING

Weeds are yet another obstacle to overcome, but most hobbies do not come without their cleanup. Weeding can put tremendous strain on the achy joints in your body. Annual and perennial weeding involves lots of pulling and tugging which

can lead to hand strain on already sore or swollen joints. To alleviate some of that strain, invest in a pair of gloves that will
cushion the hands while working. Bionic gardening gloves are
an invention approved by orthopedists and gardeners who have
arthritis, and since RA and osteoarthritis share a lot of similarities, they are perfect for us as well. They offer extra support
around the wrists and comfortable pads for gripping tools. I
certainly don't have these, but if I win the lottery, I will consider
looking into them.

Another trick is to do weeding little by little and *often*. When
you see a stray weed come up, go ahead and pull it as you go,
rather than making a small task into a bigger one by letting it
grow and establish its roots. You can also use chemical weed
killers to keep the process even simpler, but these are powerful.
Test them out on a small, discreet area before you tackle a
whole yard. They kill a lot more than you expect, sometimes.

I have learned to make weeding my "no sweat" exercise. Here's how. It's hot where I live, and even a few minutes of
yard work can leave you dripping in sweat. I have decided that
whether I am in my street or yard work clothes and I am in the
yard, I will use any random weed as an opportunity to stretch,
or do a lunge, or do a toe-touch (knees bent, of course) and pull
the weed. Often, I just toss it, roots exposed, in a place where it
can wither and die, and leave it there till my next clean up.

The no-sweat part comes in next. I do this a few times,
moving to the next culprit I see, until I begin to sweat. At that
point, if I am still in my office clothes, I dash into the house and
cool off and go about my business.

Because I manage to walk through the yard to my car, the
compost pile, to walk the dogs, I wind up doing five or six mini
weeding sessions each day—and all without changing my
clothes or getting all sweaty.

.   .   .

TIDYING UP AND POWER TOOLS

When it comes to raking and sweeping, something about that motion causes me to regret it the next day. I guess my back is not flexible enough to do the rotational movement that often comes with raking.

New power tools can make light work of things like blowing off patios and porches. But a warning: these tools can be very heavy when you purchase the cordless option. I was all gung-ho about things like cordless blowers and even string trimmers until I used some. The battery technology is great—but it can make these tools very heavy.

I was once able to use a string trimmer at our house, until we upgraded to a cordless model. Its motor is very heavy and offset by an overly long pole from motor to cutting head. While lugging an extension cord was no fun with the electric, at least I could lift that electric string trimmer.

Anything weighty that I have to carry on one side of my body gives me trouble. For blowing, I have discovered the perfect hack: the shop vac. We have a shop vac that I use to blow off the porch, sidewalk and driveway. It sits on four wheels, making it stable and it carries its own weight. I simply pull it around behind me. And the one I use is a lot quieter than a regular blower. The long nozzle tube helps me avoid too much repetitive stooping. I can't recall how I first decided to use a shop vac this way, but now a chore I loathed is one I can do bi-weekly with pleasure. (Yeah. Radical. I know.)

A FINAL NOTE FOR EVERY DAY USE

This tip was suggested by an early reader of this book, (thank you Joseph) and was too good to not include. It is something I do, and which I teach in my personal organization classes. In my classes, I call it the "Do One More Thing Principle."

Every time you leave an area, look around and do a quick five to 15 second clean up. This can be as easy as picking up a used glass and taking it to the kitchen, folding the afghans you keep on your couch, or starting the dishwasher.

The point is to do the small tasks that take seconds, rather than let those tasks accumulate until you have a big project.

I like to think of this as asking myself, "What do I want this space to look like the next time I come in?" That means I tidy my desk as I leave work. Collect any miscellaneous trash from my car as I get out. Hang up towels properly. That way, when I re-enter that space, I am met by a peaceful, welcoming atmosphere, not built-up chaos.

COOKING AND LAUNDRY

*T*his section will focus on hacks, tips and tricks for the never-ending work of two critical household chores: laundry and cooking.

Cooking may not seem like much of a chore to some—but when you have an achy body, swollen joints and unstable fingers, it can be as much of a painful process of bending, squatting and scrubbing as some of the other rooms of the house.

Cooking has perplexed me my entire life. I am a project person. I like to tackle something and just *get it done.* But the need to cook seems to resurface every day. How very aggravating. If would only stay done.

With this predisposition to resent the daily nature of cooking, adding in the increasing difficulty with daily tasks, it's no wonder I want to keep Uber Eats™ and Door Dash™ on speed dial. Alas, that is not only unhealthy, but also terribly expensive.

Let's face it: humans must eat. And that means figuring out ways to approach daily meal times logically and creating systems that help ease the burden of meal prep and cooking.

IN THE KITCHEN AND COOKING

One of my least favorite tasks in the kitchen is meal prep. My favorite is watching my husband cook.

There is nothing worse than the tedious, unforgiving process of peeling potatoes, chopping vegetables or kneading dough. I love to eat, don't get me wrong. I also equally enjoy the comfort of a great home-cooked meal and serving it to my family. It's everything that comes before that point that has me frowning with my hands on my hips as I look into the refrigerator, wondering if we should just order take-out instead.

I have attempted to compile a list of ways to make meal prep and cooking that much easier for everyone. Even if you are not someone who struggles with RA, these tips could be useful to you and save you time and energy on making those weeknight meals.

The first step, which should encompass everything in the following section, is to prioritize and organize. Yes, we're coming back to this topic once again. I like to map out my plans and figure out what is most important to accomplish first. Cooking is not just a physical task, but a mental one, too. There are time management components involved in the entire process. You don't want one dish to be done before the other—and especially, you don't want to get too tired spending a lot of time on one dish and then scrap the other half of the delicious meal you were planning.

Break down the processes of the different components of your meal, and try to have everything laid out, ready to use, and easily accessible before you start to cook.

Another thing is to think strategically. If I am moving something heavy or hot, I plan out my route and ensure I have a "landing" place at the item's destination. If you need a stock pot full of water, consider filling it after it's on the cooktop. Fancy houses have pot fillers for this purpose, but for the rest of us using a plastic pitcher to fill the pot is easier and less painful than carrying a heavy pot across the kitchen.

Remember: if you fail to plan, you plan to fail. So, make sure you're thinking through your tasks thoroughly before starting.

KITCHEN DESIGN AND ACCESSIBILITY

Just like decluttering and rearranging the living room furniture can make life easier, the structure of your kitchen can either be a hindrance or an advantage. Counter space and height, as well as placement and type of kitchen appliances are important features to consider. And if you have the means to design or remodel your kitchen to fit your needs—do it.

We had a double cabinet (four doors total) that used to require you to be on your hands and knees and stick your shoulders inside to reach the back. We had the cabinet doors removed and four deep drawers installed. We keep daily-use items in the top drawers and seldom used items in the bottom drawers. Additionally, big knobs on drawers are the way to go. We have bars that you can put your whole hand through to pull out the drawers.

Another cabinet tip is to construct your corner cabinet spaces—the ones that I find myself reaching into the back of, flailing my hand around for whatever I am looking for at the time—into a handy lazy Susan.

Having that easy, round cabinet that you can turn with a push of your hand and reach everything will save you from being like me and reaching into the abyss while straining yourself. This particular movement or reach involves me squatting (very painful), an awkward torso twist and an extension of my arm. Things that go in that cabinet seldom emerge.

We also have our oven at an unusual height. It is a built-in double oven, and when we requested it elevated slightly for me, but not high enough to make a drawer beneath it, the contractor was so opposed to it he consulted the building codes. Turns out you can have any height you want, even if it does "waste" space. You can also look into lowering your counter heights—something extremely useful for those in wheelchairs—as well as other common appliances you find yourself using. For example, our microwave is a drawer, rather than front-opening, and it's beneath a counter. In a lot of homes, microwaves are positioned over the stove, but I didn't want the risk of reaching into a microwave over the cooktop and pouring hot liquid all over myself if my grip failed.

I also want to mention here that there are customizable options for your stove to reduce the amount of reaching you do —consider a two-burner stove rather than a four-burner so you're less likely to reach over hot pots while cooking multiple dishes at once. There's also the possibility of battery or electric pot stirrers that will do the job for you. They are incredibly handy when making sauces or soups that need constant attention and stirring. And for quick jobs, an induction burner is a great appliance to use. They heat up the kitchen far less than your range, and are great for single pot dishes or meals. Mine also has a thirty-minute timer, where it turns itself off if I happen to doze off or get engrossed in a book.

Additional ways to "bring your kitchen to you," include investing in a great kitchen sink sprayer—a good one with hard and soft stream helps wash and rinse pots without holding them under the water. Get some small step stools or grabbers that will help you cut down on the amount of reaching, pulling, or stretching that you do while maneuvering around your kitchen. I keep a small counter-height stool in the kitchen to sit on when I need to rest, or simply rest my feet. Sometimes I stand on my small step stool when doing hand work at the counter, to ease the strain on my shoulders because our countertops are rather high since my husband (who is the primary cook) is much taller than I am.

Another adaptation we were lucky enough to have is one very low counter in our kitchen. This was pure luck, as our house originally had a 1930s kitchen. When re-doing the kitchen, we decided to keep an original counter that was lower than 28 inches high. This is great for me, because I'm under five-feet tall. I will admit, this was pure luck, and I am not sure I would have had the gumption to have a contractor install it had it not already been there.

And while we are on the discussion of kitchen contractors, I want to share an experience we had with several of the contractors we met with when planning our renovation. We found a lot of pressure exerted on us to do the "in" thing. For example, we wanted vinyl tile floors—I know, cheap, huh? But they are much better on my feet than tile floors. This was strongly opposed by contractors, who argued that it was out of style, tacky, and wouldn't add to the resale value of our home.

I had to keep insisting that we weren't focusing on resale value—we wanted a kitchen we would love. Another bone of contention was our built-in, under-counter dog bed. Dogs want to be with their humans. And if food is likely to find the floor, they love to help us clean it up. But dogs underfoot in the kitchen can be a huge challenge. They lie in the middle of the floor, bump you, and generally become a nuisance. So, we wanted a place just for them. And I had to argue with contractors for the right to have my own dog cubby in my own kitchen. Finally, we found an older, dog-loving contractor who understood our desire for a kitchen built just for us and our needs. And he did a great job. A dog-free and comfy floor make our kitchen a pleasure to work in.

SMART(ER) APPLIANCES

While we are discussing ways to design or modify your kitchen to meet your needs, I wanted to mention there are a variety of smart appliances to look into that may be helpful in the kitchen, as well. Smart appliances aren't inexpensive, but it can be helpful with time management and stress relief to have even one of these in your home. (As long as you have good wi-fi.)

Smart ovens and refrigerators are now controllable from apps on your phone—a path that a lot of home appliances are seeming to take. You can control the temperature of your stove top from your phone without the hassle of reaching over the cooktop to turn the dial. This also works for the things on the inside of the oven as well—lessening the amount of door opening and checking that you need to do, which will keep all that heat from releasing and lengthening your cooking time. Additionally, smart refrigerators allow you to check the contents of your fridge from your phone, which is helpful for when you're at the grocery store and have forgotten your list.

There are smart microwaves and toasters—the former can have voice activated commands, while both can be touchless.

There are also motion activated faucets available for home use these days, making cleaning your hands a touch free activity, and if you're filling a pot, both hands can stay securely on the pot.

TIPS AND TECHNIQUES

The proper use of kitchen tools will really improve your kitchen experience.

One of my pet peeves is using a dull knife; have you ever tried to cut through something with an unsharpened knife that you've had for years but refuse to throw away or replace? I'll tell you, it's awful. So, some of those decluttering hacks from earlier with come in handy. Replace old, worn-out cutting utensils with easy grip, lightweight ones to keep yourself—and your knives—sharp in the kitchen. OXO™ Good Grips™ kitchen tools are a great brand that I highly recommend, and they have knives in their lineup.

Recently, I found that pivot knives are popular among those who find their grip slipping in the kitchen. At one end of the board, the tip of the knife is mounted in a stationary fashion to a cutting board, allowing you to grip the end and move the food to the knife, rather than the other way around. Just look online for pivot knives and disregard the folding pocket knives that will also result.

Additionally, if you're looking to save both time and energy, use food processors and micro choppers for vegetables. I use one for the days when I'm just not able to pick up that knife and do all the work myself. I like to use frozen, pre-cut vegetables as well. There are also "spiked" cutting boards that help hold food in place for a little bit of extra stability when cutting. Give Amazon a look for great adaptive cutting boards at various price points.

Accessibility is incredibly important in personal energy conservation. I keep everything that I use frequently—spices, oils, sugar, etc.—in the lowest shelf in our over-the-counter cabinets. That way, I'm not doing much bending or reaching for these items in my time of need.

Here are some suggestions for your time in the kitchen. I hope you find a couple of ideas you can put to use.

LOCATION, LOCATION, LOCATION

Keep things where you use them. Sounds obvious, but are you really doing it? I don't have my baking spices mixed in with our other spices, because I seldom bake, so I can keep those in a less convenient place. But things we use regularly are kept as close to the place of use as possible. We even keep a measuring cup in the sugar canister.

Knives, Cutting and Chopping

First, remember you can buy a lot of things pre-cut, especially vegetables. Look in the frozen food section. As mentioned above, sharp knives are essential. Consider getting a rocker knife for repetitive cutting. I use mine not only on herbs and vegetables, but on things like pulled pork.

Make sure you keep your hands dry when using knives, as they can become very slippery. If, by chance a knife slips away from you, do not try to save it from the fall by grabbing it. That could result in a nasty cut. Better to step back and let gravity have its way.

One more thing, in the service of interesting statistics, the author of Freakonomics™ has estimated that bagel cutting is the 5th most dangerous activity in American kitchens. (https://freakonomics.com/2009/11/30/bagel-danger/). There are a lot of gadgets to make this task safer. Or buy them pre-sliced and use a fork to perforate them so they are cut completely.

And one final tip, watch a few YouTube™ videos on knife use. They have excellent tutorials that will help you use knives more safely and efficiently.

Opening Bottles, Cans and Other Packaging

This may sound strange, but if you have a full-serve grocery store in your community, you might ask if the bagger, or some other employee, could open (and reclose securely) all your difficult products. Pickle jars were designed to thwart me. It takes about two seconds for a bagger to pop the seal and reclose the jar. So far, I have never been refused when I have asked for this favor. I think some baggers find it mildly entertaining. They usually share stories of their moms or grandmothers with similar issues.

If you don't have access to a strapping bagger, there are electric openers for twist tops. There are also those floppy silicone mats to give your grip a boost. If you're trying the "run the lid" under hot water" technique, be sure to dry the jar and your hands thoroughly.

After you've succeeded in opening a stubborn container, many say things like "Shake Well Before Using." I have discovered that rolling the container on a dish towel on the counter can achieve the same result a little more gently.

One Pot Meals

Don't forget about your slow cooker, instant pots and other electric tools. When you can prepare a complete meal in a single pot, you've eliminated a lot of work for yourself. And single pot or single dish meals aren't just cooked in slow cookers. Google "one pot meals" and you will be amazed at the variety—and many are meals that claim to take thirty minutes or less to prepare.

Clean-up has been made easier for them, too. I like to place a liner in my slow-cooker before I start a meal, that way when I'm done, all I have to do is gather up the plastic and throw it away. You can find them in the grocery store for a few bucks, and they really are worth it.

A recent discovery for me is the concept of "sheet pan" dinners. These are complete meals cooked in the oven on a single rimmed baking sheet. Search "sheet-pan dinners" for lots of suggestions. These are a great alternative when you want a crispy, delicious alternative to a one pot meal.

Lifting and Transferring Things

When you are moving things around the kitchen, especially heavy (e.g., pots full of water) or hot things, plan your route before you start. Make sure you have a landing area. If you are going a distance, check for an interim stop if you need one. Consider moving lighter or smaller items to the larger one, if possible. You can also consider both open shelving and storage, like pot racks, to keep things in sight, and eliminate repeated stooping and searching for things. We even decided to forgo drawer fronts on our main storage drawers, and instead have just a low edge that doubles as a pull. We can see most everything without digging through drawers.

Hand Tools and Gadgets

Look for palm potato peelers, rather than the traditional type, wielded like a knife. Get tools with large and padded handles. OXO™'s Good Grips™ brand have virtually any kitchen too you need in a hands-friendly version. When it comes to fine work, try a garlic crusher, rather than mincing it. And use a potato masher on things you need to work into a smooth texture.

Fatigue Zappers

Try an anti-fatigue mat anywhere you stand for long periods —especially in front of the sink or stove top. We keep a small stool with a low back in our kitchen so I can rest if needed. I have mentioned step stools. Grabbers work well to bring light objects to you, rather than struggle to reach them.

Check your footwear, too. Chefs often wear special non-slip-soled shoes designed to keep them on their feet for hours. If you're cooking in flip flops, rethink that.

Hand Aids

If you have dexterity issues, in addition to the OXO™ products, look for special tools designed just for you. There are plates and bowls with lips on the edge to push your food against to get it on your utensil. And adding foam grips to tools can make them easier on your hands. I once did actual nerve damage to my hand when peeling potatoes in bulk. My index finger stayed numb for almost a year—all from ten pounds of peeled potatoes.

I will also mention here those double-walled or insulated steel tumblers that everyone carries around all the time. I learned years ago to only use insulated glasses or tumblers, because in the humid American south, condensation forms on any chilled beverage, even in the winter. Condensation makes things slippery for me, and after having too many spills to bear, I made the permanent switch to insulated drinkware. Enter our penchant for oversized drinks. It was hard to find tumblers that were slim enough for me to grip (and to fit in my car's cup holder). I found slim tumblers after a concerted search, and they make my life easier and neater. A brand I have discovered with a slim design complete with a textured grip is Contigo®.

Your Built-In Tools

Learn how to use your biggest muscles for each task you attempt. If you are moving a heavy pot or giant watermelon, press your elbows to your sides to engage your core. That's much easier than carrying a watermelon with the strength of your arms alone. If you are stirring or chopping for a long period of time, don't just use your wrist, use your arm as well, and this will reduce the stress on your wrist.

OTHER USEFUL KITCHEN TOOLS

If you are a foodie, or married to one, like I am, and want top-of-the-line cladded pots and pans, buy the ones that only have cladding on the bottom—not the bottom and sides. You'll still have your heat dispersing characteristics, but the pots will be much lighter.

Some of our additions to the meals in my home come in

cans. And not all of the cans have those convenient pop tops, so when I find myself having to hand-crank a can opener all the way around a thing of green beans—it's cause for an audible groan. Luckily, they have mountable, electric can openers now that can take some of the weight of that task off of me.

In addition to canned goods, my spice rack is an important addition to my kitchen setup. I used to keep all of the little individual bottles and containers in a cabinet that was eye-level, but in more recent years, I have opted for a reusable, glass set—that spins. I have it on my kitchen counter where I do most of my food prep for easier access.

IF ALL ELSE FAILS

And last, but not least, are the ideas I mentioned earlier: Uber Eats™ and other delivery services like Waitr™. But there is another option, too.

Home-delivered meal kits are becoming very popular, and some brands are becoming quite budget-friendly. These kits have much of the prep work covered and they include the spices, so you don't have to buy a four-ounce bottle of a seasoning when you need half a teaspoon. They also cater to just about any diet preference you could have.

This article in Self magazine (https://www.self.com/story/the-12-best-meal-kit-delivery-services-for-easy-pre-prepped-dinners-and-smoothies) reviews twelve different options. And when you find one that meets your dietary needs and budget, many offer significant discounts to entice you to try their service. These deliveries will let you still enjoy the cooking aspect of the kitchen but will considerably reduce the purchase and prep phases of cooking.

LAUNDRY

Laundry is another (seemingly never-ending.) task that involves a lot of bending and standing. With this household chore, I find myself struggling with conserving my energy while moving room to room to collect the clothes, then figuring out how to lessen the strain it puts on my body to get it sorted and in the machine. I'm big on sorting—darks, lights, "folding" versus "hanging," knits, and so forth. I have found this results in smaller, easier-to-manage loads. One challenge for me is folding, the clean laundry and putting it away. It's certainly one of those chores that involves a lot of prioritizing and determination. Laundry takes a lot of energy from me over my weekends, and I begrudge every bit of it, even though I consider it one of my favorite chores.

However, there are a variety of hacks that I have learned over the years that have taken some of that weight off my shoulders. Before we explore those, let's go back to basics for a few minutes.

Laundry requires a good defense. You start mastering laundry when you are shopping. If you think about laundering when you are buying, you'll make better decisions. Years ago, I decided to go with one color for all our towels. No more sorting them by bathroom color scheme. It was so simple and reduced a step. Other defensive moves:

Shopping for work clothes? Go wrinkle free.

Hand wash and drip dry? Just say no.

Fussy details that will require an hour with an iron? Nope. Keep looking. See how a good defense will save you precious time and energy?

Just home from work? Check yourself and see if your clothes are wearable again. If so, go hang them up properly to be worn again later. (Empty the pockets.)

Set aside low maintenance weekend and afterwork clothes

that you can be more casual with and put these on right after
you get home.

Bonus idea from Grandma's arsenal: Wear an apron when
you cook or do messy things in the yard. On an apron, a stain
is practically a badge of honor.

LAUNDRY TOOLS

With laundry, reaching is my main focus. I just can't bend down
and stand back up over and over to grab clothes off of the floor
some days. So, I like to use a grabber stick to help pick things up
from the floor in my closet. It also helps reaching for things on
shelves higher up that I can't get, or picking up dog or cat
toys. If you don't have a grabber tool, using a pair of tongs is
also helpful. Especially if they have the rubber grips on the ends
—then you have a helpful tool for both the kitchen and the
laundry.

Another handy tool I've found that helps me—because most
of the time, our dirty clothes are not centralized in one place—
is a rolling laundry basket. Rather than carrying it as it gets
heavier and heavier, I'm able to easily roll it from room to room.
And with the added help of my grabber stick, the stress of
laundry day is leavened. I'm slowly but surely trying to get my
husband on board with keeping our clothes in one room so that
it lessens walking back and forth on me, but alas, it's still a work
in progress.

For stains, I keep pre-treatment spray in the master bathroom, where most laundry accumulates, and try to spray things
the moment they are removed, to minimize any hand scrubbing
needed on stains. I also gave up using multiple laundry products. On days when my hands are balky, it's hard enough to
manipulate all those fancy spouts or squirters. I've found it
important to have pre-measured ingredients that I can just

throw into the load rather than lifting, measuring and pouring. Laundry pods will help you avoid spilling things if your grasp fails you while you are trying to put the detergent in.

OTHER LAUNDRY IDEAS

1. Use a good detergent. I was surprised when I started spending a bit more for detergents that made claims about stain and odor removal. They were much better than my basic generic. After I found one I liked, I eventually stumbled upon a store brand equivalent.
2. Use the correct amount of detergent. Too little and your clothes won't be clean. Too much and you can create problems for yourself (re-washing to rinse out suds) and for the machine itself.
3. Wash your clothes in the hottest water the items are rated for. Warmer water activates the cleaning properties of your detergent.
4. Get an anti-fatigue mat if you stand while folding laundry.
5. Have open shelf storage for your cleaning products within easy reach.
6. If you have the option, locate the laundry room nearest the greatest source of clothes. This could be the master bedroom, or even the side of the house where the kids' bedrooms are located.
7. If you are in a position to design your own laundry room, consider making it wheelchair accessible, even if it does not have to be at the moment.
8. If you can have a folding area, get it at a height that fits your stature. Better yet, see if there is an adjustable option. What you do standing now might

be something you want to do seated in the midst of a
flare.

9. Delegate when needed. Don't be afraid to outsource a
few weeks' worth of clothes if you've had a hard spell
and are behind. Many places do it by the
pound. You can even just send out only the
folded items, and do the rest of your "hanging up
clothes at home.

10. And this is a crazy tip, but it helps to have enough
clothes. I like my husband to have an inventory of
three weeks' worth of briefs and undershirts. This
means if I have a flare, he'll be able to muddle along
(granted, some of his outfits are a bit more interesting
than usual as the weeks add up) until I am back to full
speed. I'll survive, at least laundry-wise, until the
adjusted meds kick in.

WASHER/DRYER

Most feedback on the internet suggests that front loading
washers and dryers are easier on those with disabilities because
of the lessened act of reaching up and over to get things out of
the machine. The typical laundry space is small, cramped, and
tucked away in a corner. I've seen plenty of setups that place the
laundry right outside of the kitchen, where the pantry door and
the dryer door are in constant battle with each other as at my
house. Many apartments are not disabled-friendly, unfortunately. But that doesn't mean we can't try to make it that way.

To keep front-loader doors out of our way, there is the
option of using magnets. Place a magnet on the outside of the
door in the direction it swings, and then allow it to catch on
another magnet—if you have the space to do so. That way, it

won't swing back on you while you're doing your tasks. An even better fix, if you have a wayward door? Get your installer to adjust the hinge so that it is not moving freely.

Manufacturers now produce risers for almost any washer or dryer—which is especially helpful if you have front loading machines. It makes for better wheelchair access as well, because it lessens bending down to have the machine elevated off the floor even a little bit.

With these tasks, as with many others, it's important just to realize your own limitations. Reward yourself for the task of getting the clothes gathered and take a break. Then get them into the washing machine and start it. Take another break. Rinse and repeat until the task is done.

Something I have learned about laundry over the years is that once I get behind on the folding, I may as well stop washing, because I'll only wind up with a bunch of clean, wrinkled clothes that I eventually end up rewashing.

To the best of your ability, do the clothes folding (or hanging up) as each load is complete.

If you are over tired, postpone the next batch until you are confident you'll be able to deal with the clean laundry as it is finished. Baskets of clean, but unwearable clothes all over the bedroom are just added stress, and they make me feel inadequate, lazy and incompetent. I don't need "peer pressure" from my laundry messing with my psyche.

ONE MORE THING

I am hesitant to even mention this, but I must. Laundry is mainly the result of the clothes we wear on a daily basis needing to be changed and washed.

Some with RA might be reluctant to talk about this, but just changing clothes can be a challenge when you are in the midst

of a flare. I can recall being trapped in a long-sleeved pullover
that somehow decided to stubbornly cling to my neck and
shoulders. If my husband hadn't been home to rescue me, I fear
I might have been trapped in that awkward position for hours.

This said, for personal hygiene reasons, changing our clothes
is a must. If you are wearing the same clothes day after day,
trust me, outsiders can tell. Personal scents become invisible to
the bearer of those scents, but the rest of us can pick them up
from across the room.

If you are struggling to the point of wanting or needing to
wear the same clothes day after day, or find that bathing or
showering is overwhelming, you should talk very frankly to
your doctor. Difficulties like this mean your current treatments
may not be adequate. No two RA patients are the same, and
some treatments work for a while, but then become less effec-
tive. Clear communication with your physician is critical. Don't be hesitant to bring up subjects like these.

ALPHABET SOUP: THE ADA, RA AND YOU

*P*lease note, I am not a lawyer and none of this should be taken as legal advice. I urge you to seek appropriate counsel for your individual situation and workplace. Furthermore, I am writing this chapter for readers from the United States. If you are outside of the United States, please understand that you will have to research your own country's laws.

The ADA stands for the Americans with Disabilities Act of 1990. This piece of legislation brought sweeping changes to our communities and workplaces. I was a library director when it became law, and I recall going all over the building with a tape measure and checklists to see if we had areas of non-compliance.

The gist of the law is that it is illegal to discriminate against people with disabilities in all areas of public life—the workplace, schools, parks, basically any place open to the general public. It guarantees that individuals with disabilities will be reasonably accommodated in all these realms. There is one important caveat for workplaces: The ADA covers employers with more than 15 employees. If you work for a small company or organization, this act may not extend protections to you.

When I assessed the library, I was looking on behalf of employees and patrons—in my case college students—who would come in to use the library. One of the hard things for people trying to comply with the ADA is that each person with a disability has unique needs. One problem we found was the restroom—which we believed was ADA compliant—had an entry door that was way too difficult to open. When that was brought to our attention, we corrected it by adjusting the self-closing mechanism.

I mention all this because if you have RA and are employed and begin to find elements of your position or work environment difficult to navigate, you do have the right to request reasonable accommodations.

This is where things get tricky. Because each person with a disability is unique, the law cannot spell out every type of possible accommodation. It is up to the employer, in the case of the workplace, to work with the employee to come up with a reasonable accommodation.

So, we've established that you are eligible to request an accommodation. The next question is, should you request one?

You may have very strong reasons to not disclose that you have RA. Not all employers embraced the ADA the way my library did. And just because discrimination is against the law does not mean it doesn't happen. The decision to reveal your condition and request accommodations is yours. And not revealing a disability now does not mean you cannot reveal it in the future.

Statistics from the Harvard Business Review state that only 39% of the eligible (i.e., disabled) work force disclose their disabilities to their managers, but of that percentage, more than half of them feel better and more content at their job than those who did not. (https://hbr.org/2019/06/why-people-hide-their-disabilities-at-work). It is absolutely your decision on whether or not you do so, but there are some benefits of disclosure.

It may open up the conversation to those who, like you, were hiding it previously. But if you don't feel comfortable "coming out" to your supervisor as the first step, you can try starting smaller, with a colleague that you trust and work your way up to it.

How to Determine If You Need an ADA Accommodation

The first step is to find the areas and patterns of your discomfort while you are working. Arthritis.org suggests keeping a journal for a week to track your pain and fatigue levels and how they fluctuate. Using it, you should have a solid basis to determine the patterns within your days to pinpoint what needs modification in order to make yourself a more productive worker.

The general guidelines of the ADA apply if:

- you have an impairment,
- if that impairment affects a major life activity,
- and if it substantially *limits* a major life activity

If you can say yes to all three items above, and your organization employs more than 15 people, you can bring up your disability within the workplace and in most cases be covered by the ADA for accommodations. Definitely research your situation thoroughly before engaging your employer. And I reiterate, consulting a professional advisor is suggested before taking action in regard to your employment.

Employers are required by ADA laws to allow "reasonable accommodations" within the workplace to help you complete tasks. There may be a few hoops to jump through—they may ask for medically diagnosed proof—but if it means allowing you to stay within your field, and in a position you need and enjoy, it may be something you want to consider disclosing to them.

If you aren't too keen on discussing such things face-to-face, you can consider drafting an opening email or letter. These are sensitive topics and getting some of the major points out of the way before you do have to talk to your manager can save you a lot of anticipation and stress. If you're looking to send an email or letter, consider adding these components to your request for accommodations:

- Start with the premise that you are confident you and your employer can work with one another to solve this. Hint: Don't start your message with, "After discussions with my attorney..."
- Identify yourself as a person with a disability.
- Cite the ADA laws—the more that you know beforehand, the harder it is for your employer to avoid coming into compliance with the ADA.
- Describe specific job tasks or areas that are most difficult for you and your solutions—make sure to do some research here.
- Ask for their input so the request doesn't seem too demanding.
- Attach medical documentation. You can also wait for them to ask for it, if you'd like.

Then, you wait for their response.

COMMON ADA ACCOMMODATIONS

When dealing with the setbacks that come with an autoimmune disorder such as RA in the workplace, the accommodations necessary for it will differ from person to person. It's important to consider the daily tasks from job to job, as well, but there are a few common adjustments that can be made.

As I mentioned before, with RA energy conservation is key. One accommodation is to simply take breaks when you need to—even if they're more frequent—especially if you work in an atmosphere job where you are repeating movements, bending, walking, or standing excessively. You will likely be expected to demonstrate how the added breaks will improve your productivity and accuracy. But fatigued employees perform lower quality work with more mistakes. Shorter, more frequent breaks can be a win-win situation.

STANDING JOBS

Memories of my short-lived time as a cashier when I was a teenager is only filled with moments of goofing off, dealing with difficult customers, and the constant ache I felt in my feet and shoulders after an eight-hour shift. My manager didn't care much for our pain—for a while, we didn't even have enough mats for the number of registers we had, so some of us were out of luck after we clocked in. I didn't know anything about proper accommodations back then, and the ADA was years away, unfortunately.

If your job requires you to stand, or be on your feet for most of the day try requesting an anti-fatigue mat to stand on. If you're cashiering and anchored to one space during your shift, these are great tools to relieve some of the pressure on your feet. Anti-fatigue mats can be made of various materials, such as rubber, carpet, vinyl and even wood.

You can also try a combination of accommodations; sometimes a fatigue mat alone will not do the trick of relieving pressure on your feet and legs during the day. Try changing your working position when you feel extra tired—if you're allowed to sit at your workspace rather than stand you can get a stand-lean stool, and definitely personally invest in a great pair of shoes that help with the pain you feel. It's important to remember that the shoes you choose should have great heel and arch support to provide comfort. No flat-bottomed shoes, even if they look cute.

OFFICE JOBS

If you're in more of an office environment, you have a bit of a break from the difficulties that plague those in retail; but each job comes with its own stressors, that's for sure. In office settings, you are more likely to do things with your hands: type, write, file papers, organize, etc. After multiple days of doing so during your week, it can take a toll on the joints in your wrists and fingers.

Assistive technology (AT) can help with disabilities in the workplace, and I will try to list as many as I can below:

- If you find yourself achy and uncomfortable when using your keyboard, experiment with speech to text recognition software. A lot of people with disabilities who have writing jobs say that they switch off hands —using their first right hand to chicken peck, and then their left to conserve their energy. It's not the most productive—or timely—way to type, but it's a way to continue to get the work done and that's all that matters. I also suggest investing in a nice, cooling gel wrist rest for your mouse and underneath your keyboard, to give yourself some stability when using them.
- Sitting, although it can be a much better option for people with RA than standing, can still pose some difficulties for stiff muscles and soreness. We tend to slouch in our chairs without realizing it, putting pressure on different places in our backs and hips. (I just self-checked as I wrote this and found myself

sitting in a slouchy, "C" position, with my chin about level with my shoulders.) Sitting for long periods of time has also been known to make sciatica worse. It is, without a doubt, incredibly important to have an ergonomic office space in order to get things done with a disability.

- Ergonomic desks and chairs can be very helpful. Try making adjustments, using pillows or risers, arms or no arms. Experiment with the equipment you have. You will not endear yourself to your employer if your first accommodation request is for a $2,000 chair. Do try to correct issues in good faith before making what could be a big ask, especially for a small employer.

- There are standing desks that elevate with the touch of a button, allowing you to take a break from your chair if you are centralized in front of a computer screen for most of your day. You can create these with risers, if you are able to reconfigure your work furniture. You can also look into getting a chair that has lumbar support for your back, or a foot stool that elevates your feet to take some of that building pressure off during your work days.

- If you find yourself squinting at small print, try a bigger screen or a screen magnifier that will increase text size for easier viewing. There are also stands to hold papers upright, and screen clips, if you are in a setting that requires you to transfer information from paper to an online document. It is designed to relieve neck and eye strain from constantly shifting back and forth between the two.

- Again, if all else fails, step back from your work and take a break. Even five or ten minutes will help reset yourself and your confidence to continue on.

Everyone deserves a break—we are not working machines. Have you ever heard of the Pomodoro technique? It is great for this, it suggests that we work for twenty-five minutes before taking a break, and then an extended break after four sessions of twenty-five minutes of focused work. It's been described in the online studying community as a sure-fire way to promote concentration and productivity, so give it a try if you're interested.

Repetitive Motion Jobs

Positions in manufacturing are much more prone to repetitive-stress injuries. These are injuries that place strain on your hips, back, feet, hands, etc., from performing the same type of motions over and over during an extended period of time. These repetitive motions can harm the connective and support tissue. And it's not just industrial jobs I'm talking about. Even keyboard work, if done for long periods on a regular basis, can result in injury.

Tools such as hammers, wrenches and screwdrivers have better accessibility options for those whose grip sometimes fail us. There are tools with contoured handles for a better hold on them, as well as cushioned material to mitigate impact on working hands.

Support braces may help stabilize your back and shoulders, if you find yourself squatting and lifting a lot at work. Always consult a health care professional with expertise in this area before strapping on a brace or support belt. Used incorrectly they might cause harm or damage. When I worked in retail, we were always having to reach above us to get to clothes on the shelves in the back, and so step stools and grabber tools can be helpful here, too. It important to remember to continue to bring objects to *you*, rather than straining yourself to get to *them*.

In the event you are having issues with repetitive motions, your best bet is to research solutions and take them to your supervisor. Working with your employer, in a proactive and helpful way, offering solutions instead of complaints, will often result in a positive outcome. In today's market; companies long to retain good employees more than ever.

Other Work Hacks

If you drive often for your place of employment, gripping a steering wheel can become a tiring task. There are accommodating steering wheels that have a spinning device attached to them for easier turning and movement with less effort on your part. And driving gloves are not just for people in open-topped British roadsters.

All-terrain scooters are great for navigating rugged terrain if you work in an outdoor setting and need the ability to move from place to place easily.

You can also look into what telecommuting opportunities your employer has in place. Companies are turning to these alternative options for working more and more in recent years —as of a report released by the CNCB in 2019, 70% of all workers around the globe worked from home at least one day a week. (Think about it, this was pre-Covid 19.)

These are great options for those of us with disabilities, single parents, or those who are having trouble adapting to the expectations of their office space. Discuss with your employer what your options are and how they could be beneficial to your personal situation.

You can also look into adjusting your hours—if possible—or working out differences in your expectations. Explain your need for extra breaks and time away from your desk for tired eyes, sore wrists, or whatever you experience.

Always remind your employer that your request benefits

both you and the employer, because these concessions will allow you to be a better employee. Put your communication in the context of you wanting to be the best employee possible. ADA concessions should result in less pain and fatigue, allowing you to be more productive, miss fewer days and be a more valuable employee.

FINAL NOTE:

If you find yourself needing more help or tips adapting your workplace to your needs, a great resource is the Job Accommodation Network (JAN). They have many great articles and even a handy drop-down menu with a list of accommodations for certain disabilities and common areas in the workplace.

RA ON THE ROAD

*W*hen I travel with my husband, we have very different styles. At home, on any given weekday he is sluggish getting out of bed. On vacations? The exact opposite.

"Hey. It's six am. Let's go climb a volcano."

These are not the words I want to hear some mornings on vacation. We've had to come to an understanding that I need far more rest than he does. Thus, we sometimes have days that are very different when vacationing.

He's exploring the area around the Pitti Palace in Florence, Italy. I'm napping.

He's touring the island of Corsica, learning all about their most famous person: Napoleon. I'm napping.

He's walking into the handcrafts market after our half-day excursion from our cruise ship. I am returning to the ship, showering and napping.

I am thankful that he takes lots of pictures and seems to enjoy telling me all about what he has seen. I always give him my full attention and try very hard to enjoy his travels vicari-

ously. I never want him to feel guilty that he goes alone sometimes. I want him to feel free to do so.

Not all vacation days are like this, and I really do enjoy traveling. Mostly we've just discovered I can do a lot more if we
schedule in rest days. On a cruise those are also known as "at
sea days."

In addition to not cramming in more than I can enjoy and
giving him freedom to do things without me, over the years I
have picked up a few more tricks that make traveling with RA
easier.

BEFORE YOU LEAVE

Especially when traveling outside of the country in airplanes,
it's important to consult with your doctor and see what
suggestions and warnings they have for you. Doing this early
will save you a lot of headache—especially if you will be traveling for a while and have scheduled times for medications or
treatments, such as injections or therapy. Your doctor will also
be able to recommend foods and activities to avoid and when
you should take your medication if you'll be in a different time
zone.

You can look into getting travel insurance if you're worried
about a possible flare up of symptoms. If you'll be gone on an
extended trip, I also suggest calling your phone company to see
if there will be any flare-ups in your connectivity and service
while you are gone. This isn't the case with a lot of travel, but
when I went on a trip overseas, I had to change cell phone plans
to an international plan so I could still talk to my friends and
family while I was gone. Those international minutes on the
hotel phone add up quickly, so it's better just to be able to use
your own phone.

Another "pre-trip" preparation is to literally train for your
vacation—and if it's an epic, once-in-a-lifetime trip, spend as

much or more time training as you do researching and planning. The most important thing you can do is start a walking program several months before your trip. I once read that to really enjoy a Walt Disney World vacation, you should be able to walk five miles a day. Having been to Disney World, with my smart phone acting as a pedometer, that's perfect advice.

Being able to walk (even if slowly) for a minimum of thirty minutes is a good starting goal. And if you have access to a multi-storied house or building, start taking the stairs as often as possible prior to your trip. If you're going somewhere "old" you can expect lots of stairs. And the ADA only applies to the United States—and it doesn't apply to historic structures.

Another vacation phenomenon is standing in line. For me, standing is a lot harder and more painful than walking. There are canes with built in three-legged stools, that are usually allowed with no restrictions in most museums. These can be helpful.

And when standing in front of a tour guide going into rhapsodies about a 13th Century fresco, I have found it helpful to lurk in the back of the herd, even though I am short, so I can quietly keep walking in circles, rather than stand on aching feet.

One final tip for pre-trip preparation: be ready to embrace your status and age. Once while on a tour we had a resting point, and the guide suggested that those of us who needed to do so should sit for a few minutes in the shade. I deliberately stepped away from the bench I was near, to make room for someone in need of rest to be seated.

"Why aren't you sitting down," my husband asked in a low voice.

"The seats are for the old people," I whispered back.

"We ARE the old people," he replied.

And I looked around with fresh eyes to discover that we were indeed probably the oldest people on the tour. By this time the spot had been claimed, and so I stood for thirty minutes. But from then on I was aware that I wasn't being selfish when I needed to sit. I was embracing my forth-coming senior status. (See, I can't even admit to being a senior now—it's a future thing.)

One last word about prep for your trip. Try to spread your preparation activities out over several days or even weeks. While writing this I am just back from a camping trip. I spent so much time gathering, organizing, arranging, and packing for the trip that when we finally pulled out of the driveway, I felt physically ill. I had managed to work myself nearly to death to go have fun. I should have paced myself better. Luckily the first day was lots of driving, so I napped. Once at the campsite, I went to bed when I needed to, and let the others enjoy themselves later into the evening.

And I'll mention this now: allow time on the return side to recover before launching yourself into your everyday life. This same camping trip had us arriving home about five hours later than we'd planned. And the next day was a workday. Not only did I not make it to work, but I missed the following day as well. I needed one day to rest and the second to unpack, wash and sort and repack all the camping gear so it will be ready for our next trip.

All of this said, it was really exhilarating to go on a rather spur-of-the-moment camping trip with friends, sleep out, cook out, and go white water rafting. I only declined one hike, when I felt it might be too much. But I felt so happy to be doing something "normal" and simply enjoying myself outdoors with friends.

PACKING MEDS AND OTHER STUFF

I like to stow all of my medications in a travel or carry-on bag that I can have with me at all times. Don't forget to label them—you'll thank yourself later. Better yet, if you have room to take your meds in their original prescription bottles, do that. Some countries require you to travel with all your meds officially identified, not just as loose pills. I also (within TSA rules) keep water and snacks handy for when I need to take any meds in case I'm not at a proper stopping point in my day.

If you are traveling with biologics (Humira®, Enbrel®, etc.) that may require refrigeration, see if you can get a free travel pack from your drug manufacturer. These can help keep your medicine cool. Definitely keep your medicine clearly identified (original label) so that TSA will know what it is. According to TSA information, your medicines, their travel cases and chilling agents are excluded from the liquid limitations. And always carry your biologics in your carry-on bag.

And last but not least, your medicine probably won't become unusable if it loses refrigeration for a few hours. Some can be unrefrigerated for as long as two weeks, but sun exposure may be an entirely different matter. UV radiation can be very damaging to biologics. Read your patient information carefully and check with your manufacturer for the most up to date information. And if you need a travel pack, request it from your manufacturer several weeks in advance so you have time to receive it and become familiar with it.

Watch out for the limitations on liquids, too. If you have ointments or rubs, or liquid medicines, you may find the containers exceed the three-fluid ounce rule. So some items must necessarily be placed in your checked bag.

Although I used to be the type of person that absolutely overpacked—I'm talking multiple outfits for day and nighttime for a two- or three-day trip—I have learned over the years that less is better, especially those instances where I have to haul my suitcase myself wherever we go. I don't always want to pass my heavy suitcase off to my husband to handle when I can just pack lighter and be able to handle it myself. I have a roller bag that I use and my small carry-on, and I'm good to go.

As with any trip, do your research on the climate of the place you'll be visiting and pack accordingly. I like to bring a little jacket or cover on the plane because they are always so cold. I actually wore thick socks and a hoodie during one of my flights —immediately upon landing, I pulled them off and traded them for comfy sandals and a T-shirt because it was incredibly hot *outside* of the plane.

Aim for flowing, breathable clothing if you're traveling somewhere warmer, or bring layers if you're traveling to a cooler temperature—it's all about being as comfortable as possible so that you can focus on the more fun things about your trip.

Additionally, don't forget your sunscreen. I recommend SPF 30—or more, if you're fair-skinned like me. It's so important, especially if you tend to not be outside as much at home and you're about to spend a few days baring your skin to the weather as you backpack through Europe.

And finally, not really related to RA, or any particular condition, I'd suggest cross-packing. This means you and your travel companion each have half the other person's clothes and other necessities in their bags. Twice during international travel we've had a bag go astray. By having some complete outfits in each other's bags, we were able to muddle along until our suitcase caught up with us. Granted, it was funny to see my husband wearing dress shoes at a construction site in Africa.

DRIVING

If I am the one driving, I have to be absolutely comfortable in order to focus properly on driving. I spend a few moments before each trip getting everything back in order before I get on the road. This is especially important if my husband drives my car before me, because he must change the settings of my seats and mirrors—our legs are *not* the same length, whatsoever.

Taking breaks while driving is also very important. To prepare for a lengthy drive, I try to get to bed at a decent time the night before so that I'm as rested as possible before I get behind the wheel.

But incidents still happen. My arms get tired. My butt goes numb. My eyelids start to droop because I hit that mid-afternoon slump. I find myself realizing maybe I *shouldn't* have said no to stopping at that rest stop a few miles back—even if it was just to stretch my legs—when the next one is not for another hour or so and my muscles are screaming to be elongated for a few moments. So, don't be like me—adding on a little more time to your trip is totally okay if it means being safe, alert, and comfortable.

I like to get out and stretch when we do stop; a few arm over the head poses, a little twist side to side, and rolling out my ankles and wrists has me feeling rejuvenated and ready to get back on the road. I've also found the following tips useful:

1. Stop more often than you want to or plan to. Just do it.
2. Don't ever drive sleepy or excessively tired or under the influence of drowsiness-inducing drugs.
3. Admit it when you've had enough.
4. Give yourself extra time on long car trips. If you're planning a two-day drive, make sure nothing major is scheduled on the day you arrive at your destination. If

you are driving to meet a deadline—say a graduation ceremony at 3:00 pm, you'll be forced to keep to a schedule no matter how you feel. If you have extra time built into your schedule, you have a buffer that can accommodate rest stops, or perhaps even an overnight stay to rest up on the way.

5. A heated seat, kept on low, can act as a heating pad while you drive.

6. Consider adaptive automobile controls if they are appropriate for you. Lately I have found that driver's seats have so many more adjustments than they used to that I can situate myself quite well. But if they weren't, I'd seriously be considering pedal extensions.

7. Pillows on the road can be very helpful. Try sitting on a doughnut pillow, or using a lumbar support pillow, if needed. I'm so short I can't reach the arm rest, so on long trips I bring a small pillow I can put there.

8. Think about wearing compression socks when you'll be in a car (as driver or passenger) for a long time. The same way they make flying more comfortable, they can help you arrive at your destination feeling more rested, and without swollen feet.

NAVIGATION

Thankfully, long gone are the days where we had to print the directions out on MapQuest and have our driving buddy point out the exit—hopefully—before it's too late to switch lanes and make it. (I won't even mention folding up a map the right way—that'll date me too much.)

Navigation on our phones, and sometimes, even built into

the systems of cars, have made it easier than ever to drive to a new destination without the stress of getting lost or having reroute. To keep myself from glancing too far from the road, I like to use a vent clip for my cell phone that keeps it somewhat at eye-level. I've even seen people use ones that are suction cups that stick to the front windshield. Either works, it's really up to personal preference.

I also use an app on my phone called GasBuddy. It lets me know where the closest gas stations are and their prices—really useful when you don't want to spend time looking for an exit, or take the risk of ending your current navigation to take you a different way.

DRIVING ACCOMMODATIONS

I have added a little padding to my seat belt—you can find Velcro™ wrap-arounds on Amazon for pretty cheap—and it keeps the belt from cutting into my neck and shoulder for hours at a time. Padding also works on the steering wheel, as well. I find it easier to grip when I'm not holding something hard and stiff, so I highly recommend getting a cover that can take some of the pain off of your fingers and hands. If you don't want to buy a new cover, foam tape also works well. And don't forget driving gloves. They were invented for a reason.

If it's differing temperatures that bother your joints, some cars have heated seat and steering wheel additions for those frigid winter months. Heated seats can help relieve pain in the hip joints and in the back.

In the south, we don't have to worry too much about colder weather—I remember one Christmas, it was 79 degrees and the air conditioning was on while we were unwrapping presents. But I tend to use my car's add-ons anyways, despite the milder weather. There's nothing better than getting in and having some warmth to loosen your stiff bones before you start to drive.

I also find it hard sometimes in heavy traffic to continue to glance back at my blind spot—all that twisting isn't good for anyone. Most newer models come with blind spot assist and lane assist that can take some of that movement off of you. The same goes for backup cameras—they have changed the way I drive forever, and I can't imagine not having one in my car. However, as your car's "infotainment system" will inform you, no technology replaces responsible driving, even it if does require twisting and turning.

When driving, I sometimes find it hard to get in and out of the car. Considering we don't always drive our own and have to rent sometimes, I'm never sure if it's going to be an easy or difficult feat. There are portable vehicle support handles that you can place on the inside of the driver door for stability and better assistance when maneuvering around. These are really good for cars that are lower to the ground. If you're interested, you can look up "auto assist grab bars." I have also linked some at the end of the book.

Finally, if you find yourself in the backseat—which, most of the time is more difficult to get in and out of for me—you can install grab bars that give you a bit of leverage to pull yourself out with it. They also help with balance for getting in—and conveniently fit the side of the headrest so they can be discreet and out of the way.

YOUR DESTINATION: WITH RA YOU CAN STILL DREAM BIG

If you are worried, like me, about not being able to keep up with your partner or family on vacation, there are a few destinations you can pick that will ease some of the stress of walking and

traveling between place to place. Europe is highly recom-
mended for those with disabilities because its cities are in close
proximity and usually, the attractions, restaurants and shopping are very compact and all within the same districts.

However, most European tourist destinations are of cities
founded well before curb-cuts for wheelchairs, escalators and
elevators. Neat shortcuts might wind up being a flight of time-
worn stone steps, rather than a street or sidewalk.

Again, definitely train for your trip. And also research your
potential destination for accessibility. For instance, enter-
ing "accessible Europe" in your search engine will yield many
helpful resources, including whole site about travel options
from organizations that specialize in limited mobility travel.

Please don't scoff at organized tours. Later in life my
intrepid parents started taking guided or escorted tours of
European destinations. The drawbacks included a set schedule,
but the benefits were many, including never having to touch
their luggage, except to put it outside their room each morning; being dropped off right in an old city center, which reduced
the walking; and not having to deal with rental cars or taxis.

Another great way to see Europe is on a river cruise. The
newest river vessels are all pretty much wheelchair accessible,
you're dropped off close to sight-seeing destinations, and if
you're in need of a rest day, you *usually* get a fairly nice view
from your cabin or a deck of the day's destination, or you can
just amble down the sidewalk to a cafe a few steps from your
ship.

And now that we've mentioned my favorite way of travel, by
cruise ship, I really need to let you know how great they are for
someone with an inflammatory condition. Cruise ads always
picture young (and skinny) people partying. That is NOT the
cruise I want to go on. And in reality, the average age
skews much higher than the ads and not all cruises are on party
boats—ask your travel agent for details.

Cruise ships have accessible cabins. They usually have off-ship excursions rated for difficulty—from easy to very strenuous. And if you're in need of an early night, your travel partner can enjoy the shows while you snooze—and you won't worry about them out wandering a foreign city looking for nightlife. Once you're unpacked, you're settled for the duration. I particularly enjoy sea days, when I can have full days of rest and relaxation. Days of rest at sea make the in-port days easier for me and much more enjoyable. I really want to take excursions at each port.

When traveling on a cruise ship (or any vacation, really) I am always prepared for my husband to do things while I rest. At first this was very difficult to do, especially when I found myself incapacitated only hours before a pre-paid excursion. I cringe when I "waste" money. But forcing myself to keep going when my body screams for rest is entirely counterproductive.

Travel, when you are realistic and plan for your needs, can be tons of fun, and need not be something you miss out on. The importance here is to do as much research as you can to see what places will accommodate you and which ones won't--then, narrow your options down from there until you can come to a decision on the perfect place for travelling.

BOOKING SMART

AIR TRAVEL

Of course, there are smarter times to travel than others—although, we can't always choose our times due to work or finances. But if you can, it's better to travel during off seasons to your destinations. The tickets are cheaper, and you have better opportunity to choose your seat. You can get one that has extra legroom or pick an aisle seat to give yourself better access to getting up and down for walks so you feel more comfortable during those long-seated flights. Also check into mid-week flights. They are the "off season" of the seven-day week and often less expensive.

Europe

Off season is Europe has the advantage of being much less crowded than high season. And I like traveling in chilly weather. I feel adding a layer is much easier than being dressed in the minimum and still dripping in sweat. Yuck.

Caribbean

Off season in the Caribbean can be excruciatingly hot. But if you're someone who is bothered by cold temps, and who seeks out warmth and sunshine, an off-season trip to an island can also be fun. I've cruised the Caribbean both ways—and one thing I didn't plan on during the winter, was how many cold weather clothes I'd need for the trip to and from the balmy Caribbean.

And if you want to go farther than Europe or the warm Caribbean, there are lots of other, more exotic destinations. Start planning early, especially if you need accommodations during your flight or need to reserve an accessible room or cabin.

ON-SITE ACCOMMODATIONS

Once you are at your destination, consider renting any other tools you need. You can rent just about anything you might need in terms of accessibility aids. And companies that provide things like mobility scooters or wheelchairs will even deliver to you hotel. Just make sure you book well in advance. You cannot count on booking once you have arrived—especially in busy tourist destinations.

One final note, if you've decided to rent a scooter to keep up with your group while traveling, please put in some practice time before you go out in crowds. If you aren't proficient with maneuvering one, you can cause considerable damage to the scooter, yourself, buildings and other structures, and also to hapless people around you. Backing up into someone can snap their ankle. And scooters may not stop on a dime. If you perceive a certain saltiness to my tone, you are very astute: this advice is gleaned from a near catastrophic incident I had with a novice scooter driver. These things are heavy, expensive machines, not toys for joyriding.

I promise the day I need one, I will drive sober.

SUITCASES

You want to make sure your suitcase has enough room to carry everything you need—medications, ample clothes, souvenirs on the trip back—but don't overstuff it and let it weigh you down.

A rolling suitcase is a must, whether you're flying or driving to your destination. There are two and four-wheel options to choose from. The more wheels the suitcase has, the easier it is to maneuver and balance. There are also suitcases that come equipped with built-in seating for waiting in airport or hotel check-in lines.

One issue when traveling, especially by air, is you only have two hands. So you're trying to manage your miscellaneous travel papers, ID, and boarding pass with one hand while managing your luggage (and perhaps a beverage) with the other. I find the fewer things in my hands the better.

When getting on a flight, I like to have my carry-on with all the essentials, and I keep my passport, ID, and any money I have with me very close by. I was terrified of dropping or losing one of these at first, so now I keep them in a pouch around my neck for safekeeping. I tuck it inside my shirt when not needed. I prefer the plain (perhaps ugly) ones made of cloth that are comfortable beneath my clothes. I realize I probably look like a travel newbie and a paranoid one at that, but having these things secure without having to grip them, and in a manner where I cannot inadvertently drop them, serves my piece of mind.

Once you get to your destination, be sure you have packed suitable purses or backpacks for your day trips. You'll want to have everything you need for the day, but make sure you have only that—because the additional weight is tiresome. Also look for day packs that distribute the weight across your body, so that you aren't stressing one part of your body.

And speaking of traveling as lightly (and as comfortably) as possible, unless you are in some incredibly remote area, odds are high that if you really need something like a bottle of water or an umbrella, you can just buy one as you go. I decided a few years ago that I would rather buy water as I needed it during the day (overpriced as I know it will be) than lug water with me wherever I go. There was a point when I needed to be that frugal, but now I realize my energy is as precious a resource as my dollars.

Cargo pants are great—especially when my husband wears them. I take liberal advantage of his carrying ability. I've also found great travel jackets. Travelsmith.com™ has lots of options. When the things you need to carry are divided among lots of pockets, they don't feel like such an encumbrance.

If you have a travel partner who is fit and spry, by all means, barter your partner's bag-handling services while you manage something else. I'll happily handle tickets, passports, hotel confirmations and all the other documents needed while my husband wrangles bags. And it guarantees he won't leave me if I am holding his boarding pass.

TIPS FOR FLYING

The first time I was on an airplane the cabin steward presented me with a pair of plastic wings, a coloring book and crayons to commemorate the event. I was a college freshman so that was a little embarrassing—but it points out that travel used to be different. I had plenty of room, attendants were everywhere, the aisles were wide, and travel was, if not wonderful, at least not painful. Things are very different today.

Now, instead of trying to enjoy my flight, I mainly want to block it out.

In addition to the requisite technology (for music and movies in flight) I have found it helpful to bring a sleep mask for longer flights. At home, the lights are off, the fan is on, and the air is cool when I lay down for bed. But that might not always be the case with planes, so a good silk or cotton sleep mask is great if you're used to a dark sleeping atmosphere. It can also be a signal to the attendant you'd prefer not to be bothered.

You can't take water through security, but you can take an empty, refillable bottle for after. I like to have one handy so that I can take my medicines mid-flight, if needed.

Electronics are a must-have for me. I also have a headphone splitter that I bring sometimes so my husband and I can watch or listen at the same time.

Also, pack extra chargers for the trip. It's even better if you can charge all your devices fully before take-off, that way you're not halfway into that Netflix episode when the battery goes out on your iPad. Portable chargers are a great, lightweight addition to your carry-on bag.

If you have special needs that must be accommodated during the flight, I suggest you book through a travel agent. The airline pays the travel agent, not you, so there is no charge for their services, and trust me, they know a lot more than you or I do about flying. Having a travel agent on your side is very helpful in negotiating for accommodations.

Do plan on being incredibly cramped. Seats are about 17" wide. Go sit in your favorite dining chair and note where your body falls on each side, then get up and measure that space. Even very small adults will find themselves touching on either side.

If you are very short, your feet may dangle off the seat, causing your legs to have reduced circulation and to start aching. If you have circulation or blood clotting issues this can be very serious. A foldable step stool designed just for flying might help with this. Or, do as I do: since I am so short I cannot reach the overhead bins, I always place my carry on beneath the seat in front of me. Once we are released to move about the cabin, I pull it out and use my carry on as a foot stool.

If you will need help navigating a giant airport, before leaving, I suggest calling the airport you will be flying into and seeing if they can help you with any accessibility devices or services and how much they might cost. You can arrange to have a wheelchair provided to you, or someone to assist you with your things when moving throughout the airport and its facilities.

And one last note. I know I can't wait to get to my final destination, but I always choose the longer airport layover, rather than the shorter. Having plenty of time to go at my own pace is less stressful. In some large airports, a two-hour layover is barely enough time to de-plane, find a restroom, locate your next gate, cross through four terminals to get there, maybe grab a snack and board your next flight.

OTHER TRAVELING HACKS

DIET AND EXERCISE

Continuing with your semi-usual diet routine is important when traveling. With the limited amount of energy we have daily, a series of high-fat, high-calorie, dense meals can have you clocking out much faster than a lighter, more nutritious meal. Also, remember that excessive alcohol intake can worsen inflammation associated with RA.

Stay hydrated and carry healthy snacks with you when you're out. I like to have granola bars or something sweet on me when I get unexpected energy drops. There's nothing worse than being out with others and trying to have a good time, all the while trying to hide your shaky hands and the cold sweat forming between your shoulder blades.

Now, that doesn't mean don't try *any* of the delicious foods you've been hearing about—just be selective. Maybe if you get that extra-special dish, plan a nap after rather than a hike or a cycle around the city.

On the topic of exercise, I want to come back to a point I mentioned earlier. My husband is one with seemingly limitless energy, while I am certainly not. While planning your schedule, make sure you put in rests for yourself. Don't book yourself too tight—say, planning to be halfway across the city on bikes in thirty minutes to catch a show or meet dinner reservations—and always make time for breaks, rests, and general moments to slow down and catch your breath before and after an event that takes away more of your energy.

And when touring, there's always my (sometimes not-so-subtle) habit of pausing to gaze admiringly at our surroundings, almost as if I were memorizing them. I do this in places where I need a few seconds to rest, work through a spasm, or catch my breath. My husband knows what I am doing, but I like to think I am disguising my fatigue as awe. He will even take pictures while I rest.

FINANCES

I won't spend a lot of time here explaining how to save up money for your trip—that's inevitable. But I do want to say there are things I've learned over the years that make my trips far easier.

I try to keep a lot of small bills on me for tipping—just remember this isn't as much of a thing in some countries as it may be in yours. (Japan is one place I had a friend visit and tell me they never left a tip for their servers—it's not customary, and can actually come off as rude. Again, research is so important for travel.)

Nonetheless, here in the US, tipping for bags is usual and customary. I have taken trips where at every point, I simply paid a porter or bellman to handle my bags. Who wants to return from a trip with an aching shoulder? So stock up on those ones.

And while we're talking finances, please budget in some funds for spur-of-the-moment taxis, Ubers™, bike-taxis, or what have you. We have taken more than one trip where after going full steam for hours, all of a sudden my feet simply say, "No."

Early in our marriage I'd just slog on through, trying to enjoy myself as I began to feel worse and worse. It finally dawned on me, I'd much rather "waste" twenty-five bucks than continue to feel awful. And when my feet get cranky, the rest of me does, too.

While not RA specific, remember to take advantage of your memberships, if you're a part of any. You can get discounts on flights and hotels. Use incognito mode on your computer when comparing prices—that way, your search engine can't lock onto a certain price range and try to only show you *those* tickets.

And don't forget travel agents—again—they are paid by the airline, or hotel, or cruise line, not you, and they have access to secret codes you and I will never discover. Anytime I am spending more than about $600 on a trip, I consult my favorite travel agent.

TAKING BREAKS

With our limited amount of energy during the day, it's important to listen to our bodies and know when it's just time to stop and rest. This goes for before, during, and after travel. Give yourself time to rejuvenate—you'll be happy you did, because it will make all of your vacations or travel destinations possible *and* fun.

FROM SEX TO SOCKS: SELF-CARE WITH RA

*T*hose of us struggling with RA might be familiar with a term that doctors have coined *functional limitations*. Functional limitations are described as any health problem that prevents a person from completing a series of tasks—which can be anything from household chores to job functions to self-care, hygiene, grooming, etc. Nearly 43% of the 50 million Americans who are diagnosed with arthritis report functional limitations to their daily activities, according to a study done by the CDC.

When you have RA, sometimes it seems you spend all of your time thinking about your achy, stiff joints. But sometimes we need to focus on the bigger picture: our entire body, the place where our soul lives. We need to treat our bodies, no matter how affected by RA, with love and respect.

Some things I have thought about over the years are a bit silly but have been very helpful to me. For example, wearing comfortable, attractive clothes I feel good in. You might say, "That's basic common sense," but there are times I feel my body has betrayed me, and it does not deserve pampering. I think I'm spending so much money on doctor visits and prescriptions and I'm skipping so many social events, I don't need to make any more concessions for myself. But that is wrong thinking. I have now come to believe that my body deserves more self-care, not less.

SELF-CARE for me has taken many forms:

1. Getting rid of everything in our household or wardrobe that requires ironing. That's a task my hands simply cannot do anymore. And besides, for me, soft stretchy knits both go on and come off easier. For men there are now great "wrinkle-free" options.

2. Another form of self-care has been to invest in high quality clothes that last longer, saving me the trauma of clothes shopping. I also wear black slacks, black stretchy yoga pants, black running pants, black capris, pretty much everything that covers my lower half. I have developed a uniform that begins with black bottoms at all times, mixed with tops of various colors and sleeve lengths, so that half my outfits are pre-determined every day—it's liberating.

3. Self-care can be in the form of hobbies or activities that you enjoy. Once, I was desperately ill and had to use a nebulizer for hours each day, I discovered adult coloring books. The deal was, the machine was so noisy I couldn't watch TV without the volume being so loud I felt it in my innards. The nebulizer fogged up my glasses, making reading very difficult. But I found I could see well enough to color in between lines with colored pencils. I indulged myself with a great set of colored pencils and an electric sharpener. This helped get me through three very difficult months.

4. As gardening has become more difficult, I have transitioned my yard to raised beds and potted plants. Still wanting to tinker in the garden, I went on a YouTube binge about Bonsai, and soon developed a nice, gentle hobby.

More mundane forms of self-care have been adapting the bathroom. And I was lucky enough to inherit one of those electric easy chairs that helps you up—and also stretches out for a nice nap, I might add. And since I have mentioned it, napping is a form of self-care that improves my disposition remarkably.

For mental well-being I've kept in as much physical activity as I possibly can. I tell people, I can do the same things I did before, only slower. And when my pace is too slow, we've gotten innovative. My husband purchased a tandem bike. So, we're back to biking together.

We've also continued to entertain as often as possible (in non-pandemic years, of course). Enriching relationships are an important part of self-care.

And speaking of being together, my husband and I have discovered how to continue to be intimate in ways that don't put pressure on my joints. I hope the ideas in the balance of this chapter will inspire you to indulge yourself in ways you will thoroughly enjoy.

CRITICAL SELF CARE: DRESSING & BATHING

It might be odd to start off the section on self-care with something as basic as proper hygiene, but it's not. When you are in pain and moving is difficult, even basic cleanliness functions become difficult and frustrating. I can honestly say I have avoided bathing on occasion, because I knew that the process would be painful and exhausting. So, I stayed in my pajamas and hoped no-one would stop by.

Then again, I also realize that no matter how arduous the process, I never regret getting squeaky clean and putting on fresh clothes. Thus, self-care here is a delicate balance. I try to get up the energy to shower and change more than I simply put it off, because when I am feeling clean and attractive (or at least not smelly) I feel better about myself overall. That is self-care. It's caring for all of yourself, physical, mental and emotional. And if feeling clean helps you feel your best, prioritize it.

And if a full bath or shower is not an option, try using wet wipes. Or at least change all of your clothes, down to your skin. Self-care has to be adjustable enough to meet you where you are on a given day.

DRESSING AIDS

My dad, who had fibromyalgia—which he hated because it was "a woman's disease"—complained about how hard it was to put on his socks.

He said, "There needs to be something like step-in socks."

I laughed and said, "Those are called slippers."

Little did I know that I would one day be lamenting the same thing. I am happy to report, sock aids do exist. I'm sorry now that I didn't discover these for my dad.

Sock aids come in all different forms and materials. They can be flexible or rigid, where the former keeps the shape of the sock and the latter stretches it a little and holds the sock open wider for your foot. There are also one or two-handled sock devices with a continuous loop, or a long, rigid stick that helps with hooking the back of the sock over your heel.

There are also button hooks and zipper pulls if you have trouble grabbing smaller objects. If your grip fails you in the bathroom, use an electric toothbrush to take away some of those repetitive movements. I just got my very first electric toothbrush and love it. I never thought I'd look forward to brushing my teeth.

If you Google "dressing aids" you will see there are dozens of products available for people who need them and the caregivers who assist people. Experimentation will be necessary, as what works for one person will not for another. My father was delighted to discover Velcro-closing shoes late in life. I now enjoy sleeker-looking magnetic closures on some of my sandals.

One thing that is disappointing is that "accessible clothing" sometimes looks like hospital clothing. Although it's a slow climb, there are people who are working to make fashion more inclusive and adaptive for all of us—such as fashion designer Michael Kuluva. The former figure skater has lent his platform to raising awareness of fashion designs that will help those with disabilities, particularly in the form of shoes and footwear. He is one of many celebrities that are working spread awareness, along with Tommy Hilfiger and Beyonce.

The Arthritis Foundation also has an "Ease of Use" seal that it awards clothing it deems helpful for people struggling to get dressed with arthritis. There are baby steps being made in the world—we just have to be patient.

IN THE BATHROOM

If you find yourself having trouble in the bathroom while getting dressed, taking showers, or using the toilet—there are quick and easy accommodations that can be made there, as well. I like to make sure I have ample room to move around in, so first, I keep my bathroom as uncluttered as possible to save myself the annoyance of having an even smaller space to maneuver in.

Grips are important shower or bathtub tools to invest in, because not only can they help lower yourself into the

water, but they are critical to help you get out. Shower chairs
are great to ease some of the pains of standing for a long
time (or balance issues), and I like to keep everything I need in a
shower caddy that I can hook over the shower head. It keeps the
bottles from making marks on the tub for easier cleaning
later, and I have have it low enough for easy access. I don't have
to worry as much about accidentally knocking things over. And
earlier I mentioned soap-on-a-rope. Anything to help me keep
slippery things corralled is welcome.

For quick showers, plastic shower caps are great, especially
in chilly weather when you don't want to have damp hair
keeping you chilly for hours.

I've found that many people are switching over to refillable
shower wall attachments for their soap, shampoo and condi-
tioner—that's certainly an option, too. Amazon is a great
place to look for accommodating bathroom items that will fit
any theme or home.

For more bathroom suggestions, review Chapter Three.

Remember that the most important part of bathing and getting dressed is making yourself feel better. It doesn't matter
how you do it, just that you get it done. Put on your favorite
perfume or cologne, wear something comfortable that makes
you feel good, and reward yourself for getting the task
done. Taking care of yourself even when you don't feel your
best is how you take that first step toward managing your
disabilities.

HOBBIES

I've spent a lot of time talking about how to do the things
we *have* to do on a daily basis—cook, clean, get dressed—but
there is also the matter of the things we *want* to do. I mentioned
earlier that one of my favorite hobbies I've expanded since my
diagnosis with RA is gardening. It's a therapeutic activity that I

enjoy and have, thankfully, figured out how to make it easier on myself while doing so.

Hobbies can be highly beneficial for those of us who just want a step back from the humdrum of everyday life. I like to think of gardening and some of my other activities I enjoy as a way to decompress when I'm stressed or feeling like I need some time to myself to recharge.

Having a hobby can also lead to more social activity in your life—and it's been theorized by researchers that having social interactions can boost serotonin levels, therefore combating some of the symptoms of RA such as fatigue and depression. In short, when you're happy, your whole body is happy, too. And I must admit, when people walking by my house compliment me on my yard, I am thrilled 100% of the time. I've even created a Fairy Garden close to the curb just for young children to enjoy as they walk by.

Next, I want to spend a little time going over some different hobbies—it's not a complete list, but if you're looking for something new to do just for yourself, it may be helpful.

SCRAPBOOKING & OTHER CRAFTY & CREATIVE HOBBIES

Probably one of the most well-known hobbies on this list. If you're like me, you picked up scrapbooking (or stamping, or your Cricut® or any other crafting phase) and gotten really into it for a while. You bought a lot of supplies, you printed the pictures, made the pages cute, and then realized how long it takes to make it look like the ones you might see in on your Pinterest board.

I eventually put it back down, but I do want to return to it someday. It's another one of those hobbies that can be extremely rewarding and therapeutic when your hands and wrists are being forgiving. I also like the thought of having a whole book filled with snapshots of my life, so that's something to keep in mind, as well. The key to enjoying scrapbooking, in my case, is letting go of some lingering perfectionistic tendencies.

I have found it better to just get the key items (photos and ticket stubs) on the page and complete the whole "story" very basically and very quickly. Only then do I go back and embellish the pages. When I do it that way, I have a usable, (near) finished product right away, and if I never embellish, at least I have captured the moments I was intending to. When I try to make each page perfect before moving on to the next, I get stalled.

The bottom line: turn off your inner critic and have fun.

Here, I'd also like to segue into other creative hobbies: painting, drawing and coloring. These are all very calming activities to invest your time in. Granted, they may cause issues for those of us who have problems with our wrists and fingers, but that just means taking a few more breaks or only doing each activity in small spurts. And here again, silence your inner critic. Enjoy the process of getting colors onto your page or canvas, and don't judge yourself. It's even okay if you never display any of your work—the sheer act of creation is its own therapy.

I like adult coloring books a lot, and even if you don't feel like having all the tools to paint and draw, there are plenty of apps to download from the internet on your phone or tablet. Additionally, if you don't have the best artistic skills, I've recently come across giant paint by number kits in my local craft store that are great activities to get lost in for an hour or two. And now there are sticker books that work like paint by numbers. Granted, some days my trembly hands can't do these, but using tweezers helps. And this is a great activity to share with younger generations.

With any crafting hobby, don't focus on the elements that aren't perfect. Focus on what you can do and enjoy the process.

. . .

READING

I've been trying to make more time for this particular hobby lately. It's very easy to get carried away with book-buying though—if you're like me and enjoy the quiet, comforting atmosphere of a bookstore, beware of the extreme urge to buy another to add to your ever-growing reading list. Reading is a low-impact, low-stress hobby that doesn't require much more than your time and something to read. And it doesn't have to be novels. You can get into nonfiction, poetry, magazines— which have a vast array of topics—manga, comic books, cars, decorating—if you can be interested in it, odds are there is a magazine for it. Many of which, can also be found online on your phone or tablet, which is great for those of us who struggle with smaller print, because you can pinch and zoom.

As for indulging in a cozy up with a book and cup of tea (or in my case, Diet Coke), I love, love, love my Kindle™ e-read-er. It's so light. I like to read long, fat books, but simply cannot hold an 800-page tome in my hands for very long. The Kindle™ requires only a few initial settings, and then you only have to move one finger to read your afternoon away. And you can load up the sequel right from you chair. (Okay, that can get expensive, but you know what I mean.)

Other reading-related hobbies include writing clubs, poetry clubs and book clubs. There are in-person and virtual clubs for most any hobby, but readers and writers seem to do a great job of creating subject-specific communities. Just Google your preferred genre and add "group" and perhaps your state, and you will find lots of links to explore.

PETS

Not only are they great companions and sources of enter-tainment—I use mine as my personal therapist sometimes—but having a dog or a cat is a great hobby. Especially when they are younger, they require a lot of attention, love and care, just like other hobbies that you may start on. When you're walking or playing with your dog, it can be a reason for you to get out of the house and soak up some vitamin D, while getting your mind off of anything that might be currently stressing you.

Research shows that people with pets benefit in many ways. I know myself that our three dogs and one cat are all vastly entertaining. They also get me up out of bed earlier for business trips to the yard—and they get me back in bed, too, because when they want to go to bed, they will pace until I do the same. They add a dimension of structure to my days.

I have never said "Gee, I think I'll get a pet today." In all cases of our pet parenting, the animals are strays. I haven't even had to go to a local shelter, because all four of our pets came off the streets.

I do have some specific thoughts on pets, though—especially dogs.

If you plan to adopt your fur-baby, an older dog might be a wise choice. The younger the stray we have taken in, the more issues we've had with perfectly natural puppy behavior, like chewing (shoes, furniture, the peninsula in our kitchen!), jumping out of sheer rambunctiousness, and house training. The older dogs that have adopted us are calmer, out of a lot of puppy behaviors, and in our cases, mostly house trained.

An older pet will also give you an idea of its "final" personality. When we adopted a kitten from a feral litter, we were anticipating my husband would be getting a lap cat, like our previous cat. This is not the case. We don't love him any less, but it would've been nice to have a cuddler.

Another issue is size. My four-pound chihuahua can't knock me over.

Pets don't have to be limited to ones with fur. Over the years I have nurtured hermit crabs (they live longer than you think), snakes, turtles, a parakeet, and even Sea Monkeys.™

Serious Collecting

I put "serious" here because it's all too easy to collect things accidentally. By serious, I mean finding something that you can be passionately interested in and pursuing that as a hobby. Serious collectors are discerning; not just any specimen will do. So educating yourself about the field, researching acquisitions, and being on the hunt for a specific item all make collecting more engaging and fun.

While no means definitive, here is a list of common collecting hobbies. I have focused on small things that can be acquired, cataloged and kept in a typical residence. If you want to collect horses or tractor-trailers, and have the room, by all means, go for it.

1. Coins
2. Stamps
3. Comic Books
4. Toys (vintage, Happy Meal™, Matchbox™, etc.)
5. Books (first editions, autographed, beautiful editions or bindings)
6. Sports Trading Cards
7. Rocks or Fossils (hunting for them can be part of the fun)

You can certainly collect anything you are interested in. My parents had a collection of fire hose nozzles they picked up in their cross-country travels over the years. They loved visiting junk stores and flea markets—and found a substantial number and variety of heavy brass hose nozzles. Who would have thought?

Outdoor Activities

There are also plenty of hobbies to get into that involve being outside without all of the stress of worrying about navigating harsh terrain (say, hiking) or having fancy, expensive equipment.

If you're in a popular spot for birds native to your state, you can start bird watching just by looking out of the window into your back or front yard. I have a friend who puts out a hummingbird feeder and gets to see them flit back and forth outside of her kitchen window while she cooks some days. There's also the option of using binoculars and using bird books or apps to help identify and document the ones that you see.

And if your birds are shunning you, add some bird feeders to your yard. I've found that I have front yard bird-riots all year long when I keep the feeders filled with black sunflower seeds.

There's also the option of fishing—which at its most basic form, just requires a pole, a body of water and some patience. Think about meteorology, or astronomy. I have relatives that live out in the country, and it's very relaxing to go out on the back porch on a cloudless night and look up at the stars.

Walking can become a hobby and a health builder. Just make sure you do it for enjoyment, at a comfortable pace. Remember, hobbies are entertainment.

And now that it seems that all phones have built in cameras, I've started doing some "street photography." That's basically me on a slow walk pausing to take pictures of the flowers in peoples' yards. I don't go up to the front porch or anything, but I do like to get fairly close up to the blooms planted near the street. Cloudy days work best, both in terms of outcome of the images and temperature for me.

Biking can be a great hobby, and it can be fairly easy on the joints if you take it easy and don't try to speed up a Pike's Peak. I cheat and pick only the flat streets in our neighborhood. And if you have a willing partner, tandem biking is fun, although it does have a distinct learning curve. I recommend you research technique and watch a few YouTube videos before embarking. It can save your partnership (or marriage) a lot of wear and tear.

Camping is still something I can enjoy, although I prefer a cabin to a tent floor. We are currently experimenting with camping out of a minivan, so I'll withhold judgement until I've gotten enough nights under my belt, but so far so good. And it's a lot easier to get in and out of a van than up and down from the ground.

Do not underestimate the wonders of porch sitting. We live in an old house in an older neighborhood, and our house has a wonderful front porch. I've added a fan or two for the hottest days and have found that sitting on our porch swing year-round is vastly entertaining and a great way to stay in touch with your neighbors.

And while technically not a "hobby" my husband has introduced me to scenic drives for no other purpose than to get out of the house and cruise around our community looking for sights. It might be Christmas lights in winter, flower gardens in the spring or summer, cotton fields in the fall (looks almost like snow near harvest time), and he likes to find rural roads that are curvy and hilly. The old concept of a Sunday drive is a great mood booster. And he has gently loaded me up on some of my worst days, just to get me out of the house. Even if I wind up falling asleep on the drive, I am always happy I've gotten out.

ONLINE ACTIVITIES

This includes journaling, writing, blogging, playing video games, video chatting and simply exploring the world virtually. There are so many ways to entertain yourself on the internet nowadays. Again, these types of hobbies may take a toll on the wrists, fingers and eyes, so it's important to consider that and try to give yourself breaks or invest in some great wrist rests for your mouse and keyboard and a pair of blue light glasses.

During Covid many organizations turned to online meetings and activities. My father-in-law transitioned from in-person bridge club meetings to online games. He can play with actual people, or against a computer. And there are tutorial programs that teach novices.

With a quick Google search, I found an online Bunko game.

Basically, whatever your hobby or activity you will probably find an online community engaged in it.

Share Someone Else's Hobby

We have a nephew studying film production in New York. While telling him about my fond recollections of when the first Star Wars movies came out, I realized he was a walking Star Wars encyclopedia. And being a film student, he approaches the media franchise with a discerning eye. One of our best suggestions ever was to have him come over once a week to watch the shows (in chronological, not production, order).

He's shown us parts of the franchise we'd never explored—like the animated Clone Wars episodes—and discussed with us everything from the character development, story development to design elements. It's been fascinating.

It now occurs to me that we know several people with interesting hobbies that we know little about. And most people love an interested audience. Maybe a new hobby for us can be learning about our friends' and family members' hobbies?

Exercise

Before starting any exercise program, be sure to check with your health care provider to make sure the intended activity is safe for you. And no matter what form you choose, a tip I have learned the hard way is to start small and slow and build up gradually. And by gradually I am not talking walking ten minutes one day and fifteen minutes the next. That's a 50% increase—not gradual at all.

I have read that a rule of thumb is to add no more than 10% of time or intensity per week. This will seem painfully slow. But it will help spare you unnecessary pain in the long run. But again, check with your doctor.

Exercise has definitely been known to help relieve some of the symptoms that are common with RA—pain, inflammation, fatigue, and depression. It's easiest to start with low-impact cardio if you can. This includes walking, cycling, swimming, yoga and many more. My advice is to start with something you love or are curious about, and then expand outward. If you're still not sure, you can check with your healthcare professional and discuss their suggestions for what activities they think will be beneficial for your personal circumstances.

Exercise can also be a great social activity. There are groups of ladies that get together quite often within my neighborhood to go on walks and chat, so it's a good idea to look for more social exercise groups if you have trouble motivating yourself. I know when I have had an exercise partner, or hired a trainer, I was extremely concerned about not letting them down, or paying for a session I was not getting.

Another great thing about exercise is that it doesn't necessarily require a gym membership—there's always the internet. Pop any type of exercise that you think you might be into in the YouTube™ search bar and the possibilities are quite literally, *endless*. You can try a new virtual class or dance your way to an accelerated pulse with a low-impact Zumba™ dance video.

If you're looking to continue social distancing, following exercise videos online can be incredibly beneficial. Set up a webcam and hop on a video call with a friend so that you can do the exercises together and motivate each other at the same time.

Any exercise you do, if you do it gently and consistently, will make you feel better. A feeling of accomplishment goes a long way toward making me feel in control of my life. When I know I can walk a mile, or five, or ten, I feel like my body is strong and reliable. Granted, my pace is very slow—but just knowing I can walk that far is a huge boost to my morale.

And when it comes to exercising, I have noticed something about myself—I never regret doing it. I'll come home from work tired and frazzled, and all I want is a glass of wine and some music. But if I get myself moving, and do even a 15-to-20-minute workout, I never regret it. It always leaves me feeling *more*. More fit, more healthy, more happy and more in control of my life. And those feelings are the ones in my head. Imagine what it does for my body, too.

A key element of a regular exercise program is finding something you enjoy. I have found that if I can read (or listen to an audiobook) while doing an exercise program, I will have no problem enjoying it. Try to come up with ways to make your chosen exercise interesting and fun. My husband is a numbers guy. He likes to track things. He will set up elaborate spreadsheets tracking all the movements in his program, and then fill in the sheet as he progresses. There is nothing more motivating to him than an empty blank to fill in on a spread sheet. He can't bear to leave his workout incomplete.

If you are a news junkie, listen to a news podcast while you work out.

I tend to have books I allow myself to read only while exercising. I can't read the next chapter until I am exercising again. If a workout ends on a cliff-hanger, I'm in agony waiting to get back to my treadmill.

Here are some easy exercise ideas:

- Treadmill (buy a used one from someone who is letting theirs go)

- Walking in your neighborhood or a park. Hills can add intensity with no special equipment other than a good pair of shoes.
- Nordick Track™ Ski Machine. There is a technique to master, but I have found this very easy on my joints once I added loops instead of handles to the pulls.
- Stationary bike. From an inexpensive model from the local department store to the top-of-the-line Peloton™, there are options for everyone.
- Yoga and Pilates™. And Pilates™ machines are very helpful in maintaining form. Be sure to ask about classes for the mobility limited.
- Memberships. Joining a Y, Planet Fitness™, or another fitness club can give you an outlet for exercise and social interaction.
- Swimming. Often included in a fitness membership, swimming is a great exercise for someone with RA. And if you're thinking that getting into and out of the bathing suit is going to be a significant part of your exercise program, check out today's tankinis. Available from places like Lands' End® tankinis are two-piece suits with tank tops and bottoms. They require a lot less work to squirm into. If you can manage to put on shorts and a tank top, you can get into a tankini. If I seem overly enthusiastic, it's because I only started wearing one of these in the last few years. Why did I wait?

PERSONAL INTIMACY: SEX IS SELF-CARE

With sometimes-limited mobility, the topic of sex might be overlooked as not being very important in the whole scheme of things. But it's something that those of us with RA have to address. Sex is not usually an openly discussed topic and it seems that seniors and those who are disabled are usually assumed to be asexual, but that's not the case.

I want to spend a bit of time here talking about this essential topic that often gets avoided, because RA does not age-discriminate, and neither does sex.

SEX AND HEALTH

First, I want to talk about why sex is in important for everyone.

It can serve as a form of exercise for some couples, and a study done by Plos One suggests that it can burn up to 3.6 calories per minute. Moderate cardio is very good for heart health and blood pressure levels.

In men, more sex has been linked to better prostate health. A study spanning over ten years found that the more frequently ejaculations occurred, the less likely a diagnosis of prostate cancer in their later years.

According to an article published by PubMed, somewhere between 36-70% of all RA patients experience reduced sexual health after their diagnosis directly associated with symptoms common to the disorder. Mobility, pain, and trouble with physical activity were areas that were largely reported.

A strained sex life can put stress on a relationship as a whole, so it's important to address and understand what you can do to keep your sex life healthy. I do not consider myself a sex therapist whatsoever, but I've gathered some information and helpful tips for those who are interested.

If you're interested in doing your own research about sex and RA, I highly recommend looking around rheumatoidarthritis.net. I found a few articles by Mariah Leach to be incredibly helpful about sex, and I'll share some of her findings here.

COMMUNICATION

At the beginning of this book, I started with talking about being open about your condition to make others aware of the limitations of RA. Now, I don't expect you to talk to your family about your sex life, but the communication with your partner that you established earlier is incredibly important when considering the evolving changes to you sex life.

Be open and honest about the topics you'd like to address. Every working relationship needs this for longevity and intimacy. Let your partner know what is working and what isn't and come to an agreement about what RA might mean for your sex life moving forward—Mariah states in one article that it's important to "Try not to have expectations of "good sex" [like you had] before RA." Sex shouldn't be rated. It's not good or bad post-RA, it's just different.

CONFIDENCE AND PERFORMANCE

If it's more about the confidence side of sex where your RA causes problems, there are an array of directions to take.

First, talk with your doctor about the difficulties the medicines you are taking might pose for you in your personal life. They can likely recommend solutions such as pain relievers, lubricants, or exercises for extended mobility and stamina. Some of the self-care from the sections above are important here, as well. Boost your confidence with a new outfit or haircut —when you feel better about yourself, your sex life may improve, too.

I personally find that low lighting boosts my confidence greatly. There's a reason candlelight is considered romantic—everything looks better, including me.

Before you are planning to be intimate, take a few moments

to limber up. Maybe take a shower to loosen your muscles, or even do a few stretches. As we get older, our hip mobility declines, so a few stretches every so often can help with some of the pain that is associated with different positions.

My favorite warm up for sex is a back rub from my husband, with some massage motions on my larger muscles. I jokingly call this "back sex" because some days for me, the back rub is the best part.

TIMING

Timing is also an important factor, here. Although it might not be the sexiest or most passionate topic to discuss when, where and how you and your partner want to be intimate with each other, it's a tactic that can be very beneficial. Think about when you are at your most tired during the day—whether it's mid-afternoon or later when the sun is dipping below the horizon—try to avoid those times to get the most out of your stamina and energy.

If you don't like the thought of "planned" sex, you can try being intimate at different times of the day to see what works best. There's also the option of having a quickie rather than a drawn-out session—it can take some of that pressure off since they tend to be impulse decisions.

If fatigue is a big issue, have a frank conversation about it with your partner. I had to be very blunt with my husband. If he waits more than fifteen minutes to come to bed, he will find me unconscious, and it's safer to wake a hibernating bear than me when I am in a dead-to-the-world sleep. If he tries one caress and I do not respond, it's over for me that night.

At the same time, if it's 5:15 p.m., and I'm feeling good, I suggest he take advantage of it as the feeling and mood can pass. Again, this requires some very clear communication.

POSITIONS

Going back to the limited mobility that some of us may have, positions are another part of sex we must reconsider with RA. Sex can strengthen muscles that are used during it, so it can be incredibly beneficial for your body to switch it up, sometimes.

HelloRory.com, a website known as a "Digital Health Clinic for Women," has an article titled *Your Guide to the 6 Best Disabled Sex Positions* that I highly recommend taking a glance at if you're looking to expand your horizons.

As for me personally, I will be as transparent as I can. While I have dedicated this book to my husband, I am hoping he never actually reads this section. So here goes.

First, I can no longer enjoy having limbs dangling over open space. It puts too much tension on my joints. Judicious and generous use of pillows for propping things up really helps.

Spooning has become a go-to position, but any position that keeps tension off my hips is a good start. Once we've "warmed up" by spooning, I am often willing and able (and eager) to go on to other positions that might be even more enjoyable.

Traditional missionary position is sometimes too much for me. Scooting to the edge of the mattress while he stands is much easier—as long as I have my neck and back supported by assorted pillows.

I am definitely no expert on sex, so when I was searching the internet to find names or descriptions for things that work for me and my husband, I certainly got some additional education. One thing I could not find was a name for our favorite position. So I will be brave and try and describe it.

He lies on his left side, facing me while I lie on my back (with neck supported) and with my legs at about a 45-degree angle to his. I put my left thigh on his left thigh. This leaves it supported on him, with my foot in contact with the mattress, again, not hanging in the air. His right leg goes over my left leg. My right leg is relaxed and resting on his hips or even over his chest, knee bent. Everything is supported, so there is no stress or tension on my joints. We can both caress each other's torso, and I can be as active or as laid back as is comfortable. It's such an easy, pressure-free position that I can easily fall asleep this way afterwards. [Note to readers—if there is a proper name to this position, please tell me. This will save me having to describe it step by step in the future.]

I am not sure of the cause, be it age, medicines or bad luck, but I have found liberal use of lubricants essential. And some of the best ones require application before your encounter for best results. This may take away some spontaneity, but it is a positive trade-off.

There are days when I just can't get beyond cuddling. That's fine, too. But I have noticed an interesting thing: once we've had sex, I want more sex, more often. By this I mean, if we take a week off, say, by sleeping on a dreadful fold out couch at a relative's house, I seem to be less interested in sex when we return home. But once we resume our activities, I want it again. This brings to mind the phrase "use it or lose it."

At the end of the day, good sex with RA is something that requires communication, and being in tune with your own body. If you are struggling in this area, seek help. There are many resources online. There are private Facebook groups, and online communities that share and commiserate with one another. Definitely don't give up on this important part of your life just because of your RA.

SEX AIDS

You may not want to be seen inside or coming out of an adult store, but there are many sex aids available to anyone curious. If going to a store is not feasible, do some internet research. That's more promising, and reputable places offer discreet packaging. If buying from an unknown retailer, do check for reviews of the website, to make sure they are on the up and up. Adam and Eve is a reliable, safe website that has raving reviews on a lot of their products, so if you're curious, give them a search on Google. (Although, the promotional emails you might get afterwards are quite crude, so beware of that and searching through your phone in public. Learn from my mistakes and be sure to unsubscribe.)

HELPFUL TOOLS

I wanted to take some time here to talk about any "tools" that I use or have heard about from others. There are so, so many helpful gizmos and gadgets to use that take some of the weight and pressure off of tasks, and I want to make sure that you know about them, too.

In using tools, you first need to identify which tasks are too challenging for you. The things you do every day, but with frustration from your RA, are the prime ones to find tools to help with.

One tip on tools: use the simplest solution to your problem. Don't get the most expensive and complicated tool on the market. That's like trying to kill a fly with a torpedo. Just address the problem in the easiest, most cost-efficient manner possible.

MEDICAL ID

I always worry when I'm away from my home that something will happen where I won't be in the best position to properly explain myself, my health, my conditions, my medications, and so forth. I suggest getting a medical ID bracelet—there are great ones from ROAD iD™ that are lightweight and adjustable—and making it a part of your everyday dressing routine.

Also, don't forget to complete all the data on your phone's emergency contact app. Most first responders will know to check this—if you have it filled out it can be very helpful.

PARKING PERMIT

Although some might think of it as allowing others to know about your personal life, a parking permit can save you a lot of time and effort in not only finding a parking spot but walking into the store. I know my mother, as a cancer patient, used to get incredibly tired from just this task alone—she would be huffing and puffing before we even started shopping—and I was very glad for the accommodation for her health conditions.

ROLL, DON'T CARRY

I've mentioned rolling luggage and laundry carts but please think about rolling anything you have to move. I roll a large (considering my size) attorney's briefcase to carry things to and from work. I put my tablet pc, my purse, lunch, and any papers or notebooks I am using all inside. I have a slim, double-walled steel tumbler with a watertight lid, so I can even slip my drink in there. For me lifting it into the car is a motion that is far less uncomfortable than hanging anything off my shoulders. It probably looks funny, but it works for me, and my shoulders thank me.

At my office I even have a rolling cart, with drawers, that I take to events I organize. It's really part of a steel toolbox set, but it works perfectly for me as a rolling desk, and all the essential things are in the drawers below. And it's lockable. I used to make do with backpacks, slinging them on and off my shoulders, taking notes on clipboards. Now I just move my desk with me.

PILL MANAGEMENT

Also, if you're like me and you now have an array of medications and supplements that you take in the morning, afternoon, and night, it can get confusing remembering which bottle you've opened and put back down on the counter, or which one you were supposed to take at what time—it's a hot mess somedays.

But I found out early on that investing in a good pill case goes a long way. I like ones that separate by the days of the week, and there are even ones that go further and have separate compartments for morning, noon, evening, and bedtime pills. I suggest getting one that has a good *snap* to it when you close, and then test it by shaking it around a bit to make sure nothing falls out—nothing's worse than putting your pill case in your bag only for it to open and dump all the contents out, leaving you scrambling to figure out what blue and white and yellow pill came from which bottle.

For really complex medicine regimens, consider electronic pill organizers or a smart watch or smart phone to program reminders.

MOBILITY AIDS

If you need help with mobility, I highly suggest investing in the right device to retain your independence in moving around and completing the tasks that you need to. These aids can also help with safety and prevent falls.

CANES AND WALKERS

A lot of those with RA will come in contact with canes and walkers as they are recovering from joint replacement surgery —or, while *putting off* that surgery. You may not want to use a cane or walker, but they can be necessary in not worsening your condition. Don't think of it as a hit to your self-image but something that helps you continue.

There are mobility canes of all shapes and sizes and comfort grips—something that is quite important if you're going to be pressing the palm of your hand onto it repeatedly. Pick one that fits your needs. Make sure it is the proper height, and not too heavy or light. If you have a stronger side, make sure to hold your cane on that side when you walk.

Additionally, if you still don't like the image of having to walk around with a cane or walker, look into customizing them. Fashionable Canes™ has a great selection of canes that can be excellent complements to your wardrobe and personal style. I will link their website at the end of the book.

Walkers nowadays come with amazing features—including padded seats and baskets and trays for carrying things. These are not your grandpa's aluminum walker with tennis balls.

SCOOTERS

I also want to mention here that scooters are useful when canes or walkers are just not enough support. Sometimes the pain from RA is too great to power through. Scooters can help when doing strenuous activities such as extended walking

Some, like the SmartScoot ™ are compact and fold down for great on-the-go usage. They are even allowed on cruise ships—something that certainly gives them a boost in my eyes.

Most scooters are also customizable—you can add baskets to hold your things, seat storage or luggage racks (for the more industrial scooters) and LED lights.

LIFT AIDS

Of course, mobility difficulties don't just stop there. Getting in and out of the bed and car are two common adjustments that need to be made after getting diagnosed with a disability.

There is also the possibility of getting a stair lift if your house has a second story that is somewhat harder to get to now that you have been diagnosed.

HOME TECHNOLOGY

I mentioned in some earlier chapters that a lot of kitchen appliances can now be controlled with the use of your smartphone—this actually goes for quite a few things in your house. Both Apple™ and Google™ have thermostats that can be controlled with a couple taps of your finger on your phone screen.

Additionally, there are smart home tools such as Amazon Alexa™—which uses the AI technology known as "Alexa"—and the Apple HomePod™ that serve as assistive devices to which you can call out commands. They can relay real-time information such as the news, weather forecasts, traffic in the area, and can also play music, podcasts or audiobooks.

They are very handy devices—so much that some of them can be connected to lighting as well. I have a friend that is always calling out to her device to "turn off Kelsey's light," and poof—the overhead light is off. I can only imagine the convenience of a tool like that when you get too comfy in bed at night to get up and turn off the lights manually.

Ring™ doorbells are also a great smart home investment. I like it especially because I can see when there is motion outside of my door—most of the time it's a bird or bug, but it's handy because I can also see when the mail carrier comes or when my husband is dawdling about in the front yard. Their view is pretty expansive, also—I can see my front steps, my driveway to the side, and some of the street that we live on.

I also want to mention the use of emergency assistance devices—I know you might have heard of Life Alert® and their commercials, but devices like these can really help those who live alone and could have accidents. Also, if you have the means, setting up devices where you can call to another room in the house are great additions to your home security. Normally these intercoms are in the most-used rooms in the house—kitchen, bathroom, and sometimes on the outside of the front door for identifying guests or packages.

EATING AIDS

I mentioned my beloved OXO™ Good Grips kitchen tools in chapter four, but there are a few others that make the whole process a bit easier that I will mention here.

I sometimes use plates with a lip edge that make it easier to push food up against and scoop it onto my fork or spoon. It may seem like a small adjustment, but it's worth it when I am chasing around the last few peas on my plate. (And I can always fold up the edge of a paper plate for the same result.)

There are non-slip mats for when eating at the dining room table, too. These are great for when you need to cut into meat—like steak—and need the plate to stay still. They also make non-

slip plates with rubber bottoms now, so that is another option if you're looking for a bit more stability.

COMPUTER TECHNOLOGY

Since I use my computer a lot for my line of work, I am always
looking for tools that help me be my best and most productive
self.

There are one-handed keyboards made especially for those
who have limited use.

Ergonomic keyboards are good for those of us whose fingers
and wrists tend to yell at us after extended use—they are curved
in design for a more comfortable resting position. Some are
even split in half so that you can decide where your hands rest
while working.

There are also "big key" keyboards that have enlarged
buttons and print that make it easier to see exactly where your
fingers are while typing. These are great—just like large print
books, they lessen the strain on the eyes and can make the
process of typing easier and faster.

Additionally, if you're not interested in investing in a
different keyboard, there are also voice-to-text programs that
take the strain of typing away. The program will relay what you
say in text on the screen.

Using the mouse for the desktop computer has always been
slightly annoying to me. The buttons sometimes have a mind of
their own, and the usual shape makes them an otherwise
uncomfortable object to try and grip for an extended period of
time.

An ergonomic mouse is a great tool to have because
they are shaped to fit the natural curve of your hand better
—it's basically a mouse flipped on its side to relieve
your fingers of the claw-like positioning that they might

normally be in while dealing with a regular computer mouse.

There's also the option of getting a mouse with side buttons for your thumbs and pinkies, if that's something you prefer rather than two buttons on top.

AROUND THE HOUSE

Here I'll mention some more tools that have helped me— from fastener aids to wash mitts—because even the smallest tool can save you energy and time.

BED AND BATH

I love having gadgets for my kitchen and bath that make those projects a little easier.

For the kitchen, I suggest getting those great easy-grip tools for cooking and preparing food. If you have trouble with your grip, invest in jar openers or pop-top openers that take some of the strain and grip off of your fingers and hand.

For the bathroom, make sure you make your slippery surfaces safer for movement. I like anti-slip mats for the inside of my tub as well as the outside. I heard a horror story from a friend whose daughter used one of those in-shower body lotions that lubed up the inside of the tub. She went to get out and she slipped and smacked her hip on the edge of the tub, leaving a big gash there. Since then, I have made sure not only to never use those in-shower lotions but to make sure I have mats or stickers that keep me upright if my balance is wobbly.

Also, wash cloths are a bit of a hassle for me sometimes, so I like to keep a wash mitt or glove instead that I can squeeze the soap onto and put my whole hand inside. They also cover a lot of surface area faster and more efficiently.

Getting Dressed

I mentioned zipper pulls in an earlier chapter, but I also want to talk about a part of getting dressed that has always daunted me, even before my RA diagnosis: putting on jewelry. It's such a hassle for even the steadiest of hands because the claw hooks are so small—and don't get me started on trying to put on a bracelet or necklace when you're in a hurry to rush out of the door to an event. It's almost impossible.

I think bracelet fastener aids are a great, handy tool to keep in your arsenal. My husband isn't always there to help me put my jewelry on, but if I have one of these around, I know I'll still get to flaunt that special necklace or bracelet.

I also like to wear slip-resistant socks or slippers when at home. We have wooden floors in some of the rooms in our house and I am nervous of taking a fall someday. So, I keep a few pairs in my drawer for when I'm moving around a bit more than normal—these are also great to keep on for cleaning in case you accidentally spill anything. That way your skin is covered by something.

Also, don't forget your handy sock-assist devices when putting socks on. Saves me some bending and maneuvering, and most importantly, *time.*

Other

There are a few more odds and ends tools that I want to mention here because they help me in my everyday life.

I like to use book holders—preferably the ones that either sit the book up and open on the counter, or the ones that hook to the top of pages.

The former are great for when I'm looking at a cookbook in the kitchen while trying to whip up a great dinner—it keeps me from losing my place and having to flip through the pages with messy hands.

The latter are good for when I'm reading a book on the

couch—although moving it quite often is necessary, so I also recommend a great wooden page holder with a hole for your thumb. It makes gripping the book a lot easier, and then the piece keeps the pages from flipping back and forth while you read. My Kindle™ cover comes with both a stand and a band for holding it easily with one hand.

Additionally, I want to mention something else about my grip failing me. The old doorknobs in our house are the round glass ones that are hard to latch onto—especially if I have something in my other hand or maybe I've just put on some lotion. These can be replaced these with lever handles that can be pushed down rather than twisted. But since my whole house is an antique, I'd rather not replace something vintage. There are over the knob covers with flanges on each side to make doors easier to open, or able to be opened with an elbow. Able Life EZ Door Knob grips are one brand. Then, for lever attachments, search for a "door knob extender."

If you are looking for more aids or tools, I suggest checking out https://www.rehabmart.com/category/daily_living_aids.htm and also https://www.rehabmart.com/independent-living.html

For any item you find on a website, be sure to cross check with other websites for the best prices.

Prices vary astonishingly.

DELIVERY SERVICES: NOT JUST FOR PANDEMICS

I also like to take advantage of delivery services for medications, because some days, it's just not possible for me to get everything on my checklist cleared. And really, who wants to spend a lot of time where sick people hang out, breathing the same air? With remote jobs requiring us to not leave the house, along with the COVID-19 social distancing of the past year and a half, it's a

good time to look into which companies can do the heavy
lifting for you. Do a bit of researching to see what is available in
your area—companies will most likely fluctuate in price,
discounts and insurance coverage.

PAIN

Let me remind you that I am not a doctor. Please consult your
health care provider before making any changes or additions to
your treatment plan.

With RA, comes pain; stiff, aching joints, inflammation,
swelling—the whole nine yards. I want to spend some time here
talking about two things: topical products and heated blankets.

If you have localized pain, sometimes instead of taking
another pill, you can target it by using topical pain patch-
es, creams or gels. I like to use Biofreeze,™ an over-the-counter
pain relief cream that I get at the local pharmacy. I rub it on and
wait for the magic to happen. It works quite well, and there are
some other brands, too: Voltaren,™ Blue-Emu,™ and Ben-
gay™ are also useful. These can be good substitutions if you
have side effects to oral pain medications or are worried about
the dosages you may be consuming within a day's time.

I live in the South, so a lot of times, winter is a little nicer to
us than it is to our northern neighbors. If I'm cold, I usually find
myself wrapping up in extra layers, putting on socks, or
adjusting the temperature on my thermostat. I have found
heated blankets a good compromise when we cannot agree on a
temperature. I received a USB-powered, rechargeable-
battery heated blanket for Christmas one year and it has
changed the way I think about them. When I have a flare up of
my RA symptoms, I like to snuggle up with it on the couch
because heat can be very soothing for pain. It works just like a
giant pain patch—and is also really, really good at convincing

me to take a nap. It can also be taken with me to the porch, extending my "porch season" by weeks.

If your RA attacks your hands, I also recommend compression gloves. They are usually lightweight, and some are fingerless so you can still use your electronics without worrying about your wrists and fingers swelling or cramping. Some RA patients have suggested sleeping in them to keep their hands from balling or tightening overnight.

MENTAL WELL BEING AND A SUPPORTIVE COMMUNITY

Find a helpful group

As I mentioned in earlier chapters, it's really important to have a great support system around you during trying times. That's why I emphasized the aspects of sitting down and explaining to those closest to you your condition and what it may mean for your future interactions.

I also recommend looking into support groups near you or online, if you feel more comfortable talking in that sort of atmosphere. Knowing there are others who are going through the same things you are can be a comforting experience, and it's also good to hear the creative ways that other people are adapting to the setbacks that RA can pose.

JOURNAL

If you're still at the forefront of your diagnosis and are looking at ways to tackle your symptoms and take control of your well-being, I recommend starting a journal where you can log your pain, fatigue, and any other important cues your body gives you throughout your day. The faster you can recognize the patterns, the more likely you are to come up with solutions to address them.

If you're not much of a writer, there are also apps for your smartphone—such as the ArthritisPower™ app—that will allow you to log the same information. This is also good for those of us on the go who may not be able to take a pen and journal around with us everywhere we go. Additionally, the Arthritis-Power™ app is also a weather tracker, which can help those of us who feel more sensitive to weather fluctuations and can help us prepare accordingly.

ATTITUDE

A good attitude can be a tremendously helpful "tool" for thriving with RA. It's really important that we attack our condition from all sides, which includes eating well, using tools, tips, and hacks, and most importantly—believing.

Believing that we are not just a list of symptoms or a diagnosis or a person with *this* condition or *that* problem. Narrow-minded thinking causes us to catastrophsize our condition—as if it is unbearable, relentless, that relief or a normal life is impossible. And that's just not true.

When I decided 15+ years ago in my car outside of my doctor's office that I was not going to let RA defeat me, something clicked. What I didn't know at the time was that I was using a method of cognitive-behavioral therapy that is commonly suggested to patients with chronic pain: that accepting is truly the first step. I wanted to think about my new and different future instead of wallowing in what was happening in that moment. And that's where things started to change for me.

Even though it may seem like the end of the world, or that RA is some sort of gloomy cloud that hangs over your days, there is more to life than your condition. You are far more than your RA and you have what it takes to learn how to adapt and overcome what life throws your way.

CONCLUSION

*R*heumatoid arthritis is unpredictable. It takes time to understand the variations of energy and symptoms after being diagnosed, and then it takes even more time to create an accommodating day-to-day routine that lets us continue to live our normal lives. And right when you've hit your stride in managing RA and living your life, some strange new symptom emerges, or worse, a medicine that had been controlling your symptoms seems to have tapered off in its effectiveness.

This has actually happened to me while working on this book. Over the years I have had to increase the power of the medicines I take, adding new ones and increasing doses. Now I am being put on my first biologic. I already take a different biologic for another condition, and have been hoping to avoid taking two, but alas, the oral medications have reached the end of their usefulness as my RA marches on. So I will adapt. (Let's hope my insurance company does, too.)

I have learned to be okay with the realization that I can't bend, reach, or move as efficiently as before because of the pain. And that sometimes my days are shortened (or greatly simplified) because of my fatigue.

I have learned that sometimes gathering with friends and family, going out and traveling, or even moving around my house takes a lot more planning and executing than it used to. And that's okay as well.

I have learned that the seemingly irrelevant tools I may have passed by in the store before—sock aids, easy-grip gardening tools, step stools, rolling carts and laundry baskets—are now ones that I need on a daily basis to continue accomplishing my routines.

BUT. And this is a huge "But," I am still living a crazy, fun, creative and productive life. I have found new or modified hobbies. I travel, hike and camp with rest days. I bike, garden, walk my dogs, and try to be as active as I can. Generally, all of this is done at a snail's pace, but who cares?

With just a little tweaking—and maybe a few extra naps—I can still accomplish all the tasks that I need, want, and have to. It's a matter of realizing that this may be the "new" normal, but that doesn't mean that I can't make it a good one.

My life does not feel limited. It's different, that's all. Slower. More deliberate.

I am still learning how to listen to my body's cues—it's a never-ending conversation, but one that I intend to take in stride for the rest of my life. I don't know what tomorrow will bring for me, but I know I have built a handy repertoire of information and tips that can help me.

I hope that by sharing some of that information in this book, I have helped others out there like me—those who have RA, those who have other autoimmune disorders, or even those who may not have a disorder themselves, but are looking for information so that they can help another.

If you would like to join our community for more information or if you have any further questions, or a tip that wasn't mentioned here, please join us at Inflammation Connection on Facebook. It's a private group and I am inviting you to join.

Additionally, if you enjoyed this book, please give it a rating or review on Amazon. I would love to hear your thoughts or if any of the hacks helped you.

RESOURCES

*I*f you happen to be reading this in print, or on a device that does not let you easily follow links, please email me for a copy of these listings with clickable links. You can contact me at helen@pkm.media or helenwardday@gmail.com.

No-one should have to type excessively long URLs.

CHAPTER ONE:

https://healthline.com

https://creakyjoints.org/living-with-arthritis/frustrations-invisible-disability

https://creakyjoints.org/living-with-arthritis/explain-rheumatoid-arthritis-to-others/

https://www.huffpost.com/entry/living-with-invisible-illness_b_937234

https://www.invisibledisabilityproject.org

https://www.healthline.com/health/rheumatoid-arthritis/ra-vs-oa

https://www.facebook.com/
groups/inflammationconnection
https://www.arthritis.org
https://carlascorner.wordpress.com
https://chroniceileen.com
https://www.arthriticchick.com

CHAPTER TWO:
https://www.webmd.com/rheumatoid-arthritis/ra-fight-
fatigue
https://www.ncbi.nlm.nih.gov/books/NBK384467/
https://simplelionheartlife.com/decluttering-for-self-care/
https://www.verywellhealth.com/arthritis-living-with-
4158513
declutter-and-organize-your-home-seniors-special-needs
https://www.nytimes.com/2011/08/21/magazine/do-you-
suffer-from-decision-fatigue.html
https://www.mayoclinic.org/diseases-conditions/
rheumatoid-arthritis/symptoms-causes/syc-20353648
https://www.yourstoragefinder.com/declutter-and-
organize-your-home-seniors-special-needs

CHAPTER THREE:
https://www.chronicmom.com/2017/02/5-tips-for-
cleaning-with-chronic-pain.html/
https://www.orlandosentinel.com/news/os-xpm-1993-12-
23-9312210303-story.html
https://cerebralpalsyscotland.org.uk/disability-life-hacks/
https://www.bathingsolutions.co.uk/blog/inspiration/
cleaning-hacks/
https://earlybirdmom.com/housework-chronic-illness/

https://www.onegoodthingbyjillee.com/9-ways-to-make-cleaning-less-painful/

https://themighty.com/2017/09/cleaning-products-easy/

https://themighty.com/2017/07/hacks-tips-cleaning-chronic-illness/

https://sixtyandme.com/11-life-hacks-for-when-you-find-yourself-temporarily-disabled/

https://www.hoveround.com/articles/spring-cleaning-tips-for-seniors

https://www.yourstoragefinder.com/declutter-and-organize-your-home-seniors-special-needs

http://www.disabilityhacker.com/

https://multiplesclerosis.net/living-with-ms/cleaning-tips/

https://mageerehab.jeffersonhealth.org/blog_post/tricks-of-the-trade-easy-life-hacks-for-people-with-disabilities/

https://www.disabled-world.com/assistivedevices/household/tips/

https://fedupwithfatigue.com/cleaning-with-fibromyalgia/

https://www.mumsnet.com/Talk/housekeeping/3421333-A-gentle-cleaning-thread-for-those-with-mobility-problems-and-or-disabilities

https://www.ageukmobility.co.uk/mobility-news/article/tips-for-keeping-on-top-of-your-housework

https://www.ability411.ca/answer/long-reach-cleaning-tools-what-products-will-help-me-clean-the-house-despite-my-limited-mobility

https://kickingitwithkelly.com/home/how-to-prevent-back-pain-when-cleaning-the-house/

https://www.reddit.com/r/disability/comments/4fcow6/life_hacks_for_people_with_disability/

https://www.bathingsolutions.co.uk/blog/inspiration/cleaning-hacks/

https://www.pinterest.com/disabledbath/disabled-bathroom-designs/

https://www.pinterest.co.uk/fiot84/disability-life-hacks/

https://www.familyhandyman.com/list/20-bathroom-storage-hacks/

https://www.pinterest.com/michael5115/wheelchair-accessible-closets/

https://pnwmg.org/garden-info/gardening-with-disabilities/

https://www.gardeningknowhow.com/special/accessible/gardening-with-disabilities.htm

https://www.hgtv.com/outdoors/gardens/planting-and-maintenance/accessible-gardening-techniques

https://www.flowerpotman.com/gardening-for-the-elderly-and-disabled/

https://www.carryongardening.org.uk/top-tips-for-disabled-gardeners.aspx

https://riseservicesinc.org/the-benefits-of-gardening-for-people-with-disabilities/

http://www.cityfarmer.org/disablegard67.html

https://garden.org/learn/articles/view/3431/

https://www.verywellhealth.com/gardening-with-disabilities-1094600

https://themighty.com/2018/08/gardening-illness-disability/

https://www.pinterest.com/afternoonnapper/gardening-with-a-disability/

https://bestmobilityaids.com/best-gardening-tools-for-seniors/

https://nmeda.org/disability-gardening-tips/

https://www.bathingsolutions.co.uk/blog/inspiration/cleaning-hacks/

https://www.chronicillnesswarriorlife.com/chronic-illness-cleaning-hacks/

https://www.rollingwithoutlimits.com/view-post/House-cleaning-and-Disability-Limitations

https://earlybirdmom.com/housework-chronic-illness/
https://themighty.com/2017/09/cleaning-products-easy/

CHAPTER FOUR:

https://www.verywellhealth.com/household-cleaning-products-for-people-with-arthritis-190036

https://www.quora.com/What-are-the-best-laundry-hacks-for-disabled-adults

https://blog.thewrightstuff.com/no-limits-in-the-kitchen-cooking-with-limited-mobility/

https://spoonuniversity.com/lifestyle/why-people-with-disabilities-dont-cook-but-should

https://thetakeout.com/navigating-disability-in-the-kitchen-is-all-about-findi-1840924440

https://www.myrecipes.com/community/how-cooking-culture-excludes-disabilties

https://www.disabled-world.com/fitness/cooking/

https://www.npr.org/sections/thesalt/2015/10/21/448971281/cooking-with-disabilities-an-exercise-in-creative-problem-solving

https://www.rollingwithoutlimits.com/view-post/Cooking-from-a-Wheelchair-6-Adaptive-Hacks

https://www.disabilityaids.co.nz/resources/disabled-kitchen-advice/enjoying-cooking-disability/

https://www.thekitchn.com/cooking-with-a-physical-disability-171416

https://www.iaccess.life/cooking-tips-for-people-with-disabilities/

https://www.apartmenttherapy.com/ikea-hacks-funiture-disabilities-accessibility-267834

https://www.pinterest.com/susie3273/kitchens-for-the-disabled/

https://blog.easterseals.com/16-ways-to-make-your-kitchen-more-accessible/

https://rheumatoidarthritisliving.com/adaptive-cutting-boards/

https://www.quora.com/What-are-the-best-laundry-hacks-for-disabled-adults

https://www.rollingwithoutlimits.com/view-post/House-cleaning-and-Disability-Limitations

CHAPTER FIVE:

https://hiring.monster.com/employer-resources/workforce-management/diversity-in-the-workplace/workplace-disability/

https://hbr.org/2019/06/why-people-hide-their-disabilities-at-work

https://employment.findlaw.com/employment-discrimination/ada-disabilities-your-rights-as-an-employee.html

https://resumelab.com/job-search/jobs-for-workers-with-disabilities

https://abilitynet.org.uk/news-blogs/ten-tech-hacks-help-disabled-people-working-home

https://www.yahoo.com/now/3-lupus-life-hacks-keeping-220811967.html

https://www.hireright.com/blog/contingent-workforce/7-tips-and-hacks-for-building-a-smooth-running-telecommuting-program

https://www.themuse.com/advice/if-when-how-disclose-invisible-disability-at-work

https://choosework.ssa.gov/blog/2017-08-21-using-assistive-technology-in-the-workplace

https://askjan.org

https://www.eeoc.gov/laws/guidance/enforcement-guidance-reasonable-accommodation-and-undue-hardship-under-ada#types

https://askearn.org/topics/laws-regulations/americans-with-disabilities-act-ada/reasonable-accommodations/

https://askjan.org/solutions/Stand-lean-Stools.cfm

https://www.webmd.com/rheumatoid-arthritis/features/ra-work-accommodations

https://www.arthritis.org/health-wellness/healthy-living/daily-living/work-life-balance/working-when-you-have-arthritis

https://www.thehealthy.com/arthritis/manage-arthritis-desk-job/

https://www.webmd.com/lung/news/20210115/do-blue-light-glasses-work

https://todoist.com/productivity-methods/pomodoro-technique

https://www.thedrive.com/reviews/27072/best-steering-wheel-knobs

Chapter Six:

https://polyclinic.com/blog/traveling-rheumatoid-arthritis

https://upgradedpoints.com/air-travel-with-a-disability/

https://www.arthritis.org/health-wellness/healthy-living/daily-living/life-hacks-tips/8-tips-for-pain-free-travel

https://www.healthgrades.com/right-care/rheumatoid-arthritis/10-tips-for-traveling-with-rheumatoid-arthritis

https://www.tripadvisor.com/ShowTopic-g1-i12336-k2934009-Tips_for_stress_free_travel_with_limited_mobility-Traveling_With_Disabilities.html

https://www.tripadvisor.com/ShowTopic-g1-i12336-k2934009-Tips_for_stress_free_travel_with_limited_mobility-Traveling_With_Disabilities.html

https://maidstr.com/low-mobility-guide-cleaning-home/

https://www.rollingwithoutlimits.com/view-post/Money-Saving-Tips-For-Managing-Limited-Mobility

https://www.travelstride.com/blog/tips-for-traveling-with-limited-mobility

https://freedommobilitysolutions.com/tips-for-better-summer-mobility/

https://askthepilot.com/how-to-speak-airline/

https://theculturetrip.com/north-america/articles/accessible-and-disability-friendly-travel-destinations-around-the-world/

https://travelpro.com/pages/2-wheel-vs-4-wheel-luggage

https://www.webmd.com/rheumatoid-arthritis/features/travel-pain-free

CHAPTER SEVEN:

https://www.huffpost.com/entry/fashion-for-people-with-arthritis-and-other-painful_b_58c6eddde4b022817b2915d4

https://rheumatoidarthritis.net/living/complications-of-getting-dressed/

https://rheumatoidarthritis.net/living/hacks-for-looking-good-feeling-good/

https://www.healthline.com/health/rheumatoid-arthritis/life-hacks-managing-ra#1

https://www.sharecare.com/health/living-with-arthritis/what-clothes-easier-wear-arthritis

https://msfocusmagazine.org/Magazine/Magazine-Items/Posted/Laughing-Your-Way-to-Improved-Immunity

https://www.disabled-world.com/entertainment/hobby/

https://www.reddit.com/r/disability/comments/5mzcgq/hobbies_that_help_you_cope/

https://scootaround.com/en/27-fun-hobbies-for-wheelchair-users-that-arent-basketball

https://confinedtosuccess.com/great-things-to-do-when-you-are-disabled-and-bored/

https://ask.metafilter.com/337057/Hobby-ideas-for-my-disabled-mom

https://blog.ioaging.org/activities-wellness/hobbies-for-seniors-with-arthritis-modifying-old-interests-or-trying-something-new/

https://www.hellorory.com/roar/disabled-sex/

https://www.betterhealth.vic.gov.au/health/ServicesAndSupport/disability-and-sexuality

https://www.disability.illinois.edu/sexuality-resources

https://www.everydayhealth.com/rheumatoid-arthritis/guide/

https://www.umh.org/assisted-independent-living-blog/fitness-tips-for-seniors-with-limited-mobility

https://www.healthmarkets.com/resources/wellness/best-exercise-routines-for-people-with-limited-mobility/

https://www.disability.illinois.edu/sexuality-resources

https://creakyjoints.org/support/michael-kuluva-virtual-fashion-show-event/

https://www.arthritis.org/partnership/ease-of-use

https://www.uksmobility.co.uk/blog/2017/11/arthritis-activities-hobbies/

https://www.mayoclinic.org/diseases-conditions/rheumatoid-arthritis/in-depth/rheumatoid-arthritis-exercise/art-20096222

https://rheumatoidarthritis.net/living/expert-advice-for-improving-your-sex-life-with-ra

https://rheumatoidarthritis.net/living/that-thing-no-one-talks-about

https://www.hellorory.com/roar/disabled-sex/

https://www.disability.illinois.edu/sexuality-resources

. . .

CHAPTER EIGHT:

https://creakyjoints.org/living-with-arthritis/arthritis-morning-routine-hacks/ https://www.practicalpainmanagement.com/treatments/complementary/biobehavioral/5-coping-skills-every-chronic-pain-patient-needs

https://www.rehabmart.com/category/daily_living_aids.htm

https://www.rehabmart.com/independent-living.html

https://www.everydayhealth.com/rheumatoid-arthritis/learning-love-cane-when-you-have-rheumatoid-arthritis/

http://www.lifealert.com

https://www.rehabmart.com/category/daily_living_aids.htm

https://www.rehabmart.com/independent-living.html

LINKS TO ITEMS MENTIONED

CHAPTER THREE:

BISSEL FEATHERWEIGHT VACUUM: https://www.bissell.com/featherweight-lightweight-stick-vacuum-2033.html

ROOMBA: https://www.irobot.com/roomba

SCRUBBING BUBBLES: https://www.scrubbingbubbles.com/en-us

WROUGHT IRON POT ORGANIZER: Amazon

REVERE COPPER CLAD POT SET: Amazon

CLOROX TOILET TABLETS: https://www.walmart.com/ip/Clorox-Ultra-Clean-Toilet-Tablets-Bleach-3-5-Ounces-Each-4-Count/23619934

MATCC SHOWER SCRUBBER: https://www.matcc.company/42-Shower-Scrubber-Brush-Cleaner-with-Extendable-Long-Handle-2-PCS-p-402005.html

OXO EXTENDABLE SCRUBBER: https://www.oxo.com/extendable-tub-tile-scrubber.html

FOAM GRIP TUBING: Amazon

ANTI-SLIP TAPE: https://www.uline.com/Product/Detail/S-23628/Anti-Slip-Tape/Anti-Slip-Tape-4-x-60-White?pricode=WB0761&gadtype=pla&id=S-23628&gclid=Cj0KCQjw2tCGBhCLARIsABJGmZ5vVARlNECxEuLmEqChHfNy1zXzdTvXA5ioy8oEHNUiEyFPB5R1moQaAlxoEALw_wcB&gclsrc=aw.ds

MORE ANTI-SLIP TAPE: Amazon

BED MADEEZ BED MAKER: Amazon

AMAZON SHEET RISER: Amazon

BIONIC GARDENING GLOVES: https://www.bionicgloves.com/all-products/gardening

SHOP VAC: https://www.shopvac.com/category/shop-vac-products

CHAPTER FOUR:

OXO KITCHEN TOOLS: https://www.oxo.com

PIVOT KNIFE: Amazon

ADAPTIVE CUTTING BOARD: Amazon

BELLMAN'S ELECTRONIC JAR OPENER: Amazon

REGENT MULTI-PURPOSE JAR GRIPPER: Amazon

CHAPTER FIVE:

ANTI-FATIGUE MATS: Amazon
https://www.homedepot.com/b/Flooring-Rugs-Mats/Anti-Fatigue/N-5yc1vZc9a5Z1z0scrd?storeSelection=

BEST STAND/LEAN STOOLS: https://www.startstanding.org/standing-desks/best-chairs-stools/#what

ONE-HANDED KEYBOARDS: https://www.amazon.com/one-handed-keyboard/s?k=one+handed+keyboard

BEST WRIST RESTS: https://nerdtechy.com/best-keyboard-wrist-rests

BEST STANDING DESKS: https://www.techradar.com/news/best-standing-desk

ERGONOMIC OFFICE CHAIRS: https://nymag.com/strategist/article/best-ergonomic-office-chairs.html

UNDER DESK FOOT RESTS: https://www.amazon.com/Office-Footrests/b?ie=UTF8&node=1069198

BEST BLUE LIGHT GLASSES: https://www.forbes.com/sites/forbes-personal-shopper/2021/02/19/best-blue-light-blocking-glasses/?sh=f76140713ed4

SCREEN MAGNIFIERS: https://www.amazon.com/laptop-screen-magnifier/s?k=laptop+screen+magnifier

https://www.amazon.com/computer-screen-magnifier/s?k=computer+screen+magnifier

STEERING WHEEL SPINNER: https://www.thedrive.com/reviews/27072/best-steering-wheel-knobs

ALL-TERRAIN SCOOTERS: https://www.mobilityscootersdirect.com/mobility-scooters/off-road-mobility-scooters.html

CELL PHONE CRADLES: https://www.amazon.com/Best-Sellers-Cell-Phone-Automobile-Cradles/zgbs/wireless/7072562011

SEAT BELT PADS: https://www.walmart.com/c/kp/seat-belt-shoulder-strap-pads

PADDED STEERING WHEEL COVERS: https://www.amazon.com/padded-steering-wheel-cover/s?k=padded+steering+wheel+cover

https://www.autoguide.com/products/top-10-steering-wheel-covers

AUTO ASSIST GRAB BAR: Amazon

BEST SLEEP MASKS : https://upgradedpoints.com/travel/best-sleep-masks-for-travel/

SOCK AIDS: https://www.arthritissupplies.com/arthritis-sock-aids.html

SHOWER CHAIRS/GRAB BARS: https://www.walmart.
com/browse/health/shower-
chairs/976760_1005860_1230858_4152217_2765977

SHOWER DISPENSERS: https://www.amazon.com/Best-
Sellers-Home-Kitchen-Bathroom-Shower-Dispensers/zgbs/
home-garden/13749791

KINDLE PAPERWHITE: Amazon

NORDIC CLASSIC PRO SKIER: https://www.nordictrack.
com/skiers/nordictrack-classic-pro-skier

LANDS' END TANKINIS: https://www.landsend.com/
shop/womens-tankini-tops-swimsuit-swimsuits/S-xfh-xez-
y5c-xhd-y9j-xec

MEDICAL ID BRACELET: https://www.roadid.com/pages/
choose-your-wrist-style

BEST PILL CASES: https://www.amazon.com/Best-Sellers-
Health-Personal-Care-Pill-Cases/zgbs/hpc/3764251

BIOFREEZE: https://www.biofreeze.com

VOLTAREN: https://www.voltarengel.com/what-is-
voltaren/

BLUE-EMU: https://www.blue-emu.com

BENGAY: https://www.bengay.com

BEST BED HEATING TOOLS: https://www.
nosleeplessnights.com/heated-mattress-pads-review/

BEST COMPRESSION GLOVES: https://www.
verywellhealth.com/best-arthritis-gloves-2552025

BEST MEDICAL ALERT SYSTEMS: https://www.health.
com/health-reviews/the-best-medical-alert-systems

BEST INTERCOM SYSTEMS: https://www.
betterhomeguides.com/appliances/best-wireless-home-
intercom-system/

LIP EDGE PLATES: https://www.amazon.com/plate-lip-
edge/s?k=plate+with+lip+edge

SMART SCOOT SCOOTERS: https://www.s-martscoot.com

BEST ANTI-SLIP MATS: https://www.thespruce.com/best-non-slip-bath-mats-5084877

WASH CLOTH MITT: https://www.amazon.com/washcloth-mitt-Beauty-Personal-Care/s?k=washcloth+mitt&rh=n%3A3760911

BRACELET FAIRY FASTENER: https://fairyfastener.com/product/bracelet-fairy-new/

WOODEN BOOK HOLDER: Amazon

BOOK STAND AND HOLDER: https://www.amazon.com/Cookbook-Stands-Recipe-Holders/b?ie=UTF8&node=3737111

LEVER HANDLES: https://www.homedepot.com/b/Hardware-Door-Hardware-Door-Lever-Handles/N-5yc1vZc28z

Printed in Great Britain
by Amazon

14078532R00099